Fuel
Your Fire

Fuel Your Fire

Secrets to Living Your Healthiest Life

Rosann Cunningham, INHC, NASM - CPT

Foreword by Molly Mercer, CFO
Slippery Rock University, Fellow Badass

Fuel Your Fire:
Secrets to Living Your Healthiest Life
By Rosann Cunningham, INHC, NASM-CPT

© 2019 by Rosann Cunningham, INHC, NASM-CPT

Cover Design by Amber Schoener
Professional Photos of Rosann Cunningham by Willa J. Photography
Professional Editing by Lee Caleca
Interior Design and Layout by Maureen Cutajar at GoPublished.com

ISBN-13: 978-1-7341611-0-6

Printed in the United States of America

This book is dedicated to my beautiful mother,
no doubt my greatest fan!

Mom always said to me, "Rosann, you can do anything you want.
Just set your mind to it, and go do it!" It was her words, her work
ethic, and her unconditional love that kindled my inner fire, and
my very stubborn, support-me-or-get-the-hell-out-of-my-way
attitude around my big, hairy, audacious goals.

I love you and miss you like crazy, Mom!

Acknowledgements

Thank you to everyone who offered encouragement, ideas, accountability, and uninterrupted time for this project to come to life. I am forever grateful to those of you who assisted with peer reviews, editing, graphics, and more!

Thank you to Brenda for your unconditional love, support, and friendship during the hardest year of my life. I don't know how I would have survived it without you, girl! I love you!

To Faith and Abby, thank you for cheering me on that last hard week of writing this manuscript. You put up with so much crankiness and countless hours of your mama typing away feverishly. I am so proud of the beautiful young ladies you are both becoming, and I love you to the end of the universe and back... infinity!

To my dear dad, you have been and always will be my greatest hero. Thank you so much for your unconditional love, encouragement, support, and wisdom. I love our long chats about business, sales, marketing, and life. You always have a way of making me laugh, and inspiring me to be my best self. I don't know what I would do without you. I love you so much, and I love knowing no matter what I need, you're always there for me.

Thank you to my growing tribe of clients who trust me to be their health coach and personal trainer, but who also invite me into their lives as a friend. I love you all, and I wouldn't be able to do any of this without you!

And finally, to Steve… your love fuels my fire like never before. I love you and appreciate you more than words could ever say. Thank you for the countless smiles, for the badass adventures, for your constant encouragement and push, and for showing me what love is supposed to feel like.

Foreword

If you're opening this book, chances are that you are searching for answers. Perhaps answers to why you are gaining weight, why you have lost your energy, why you have symptoms like stomach problems or chronic headaches that you can't get under control, why stress is affecting you more than in the past, and perhaps why you are just feeling "off".

A year ago, that was me.

Although my career was thriving and I was doing a decent job balancing work with motherhood and marriage, something was off. I had gained 25 pounds and counting in the past three years, which on a 5'2" frame was nothing I could hide. My demanding life made cooking and nutrition take a backseat. Exercise was sporadic at best. And while these patterns and habits were similar to those I had throughout my 20's and 30's, it was as if everything was catching up to me all at once. I was often dealing with nagging headaches, stomach issues, or fatigue. My career and family commitments require me to bring my A-game, which was getting harder and harder to do. I was starting to feel like a stranger in my own body.

In November 2018, my path crossed Rosann's on a Saturday night at the wine bar in our small town. What stuck out to me was the vitality that she had, a smile that lit up a room, infectious enthusiasm, and she was fit and strong… with a glass of wine in her hand… which I thought was awesome for a health coach! We only briefly chatted, but the encounter stuck with me. It was as if she embodied the polar opposite of how I was feeling about my health at that time in my life. While I had some hesitations, I followed the spiritual nudge I had to pursue this and took a leap of faith. I reached out to Rosann and signed on as a client.

I had started and quit other programs in those past few years trying to find that silver bullet. I had great intentions but would always drift and eventually quit. It hadn't worked because I tend to prefer to be in control and do things my own way, and also because they never seemed to mesh with my lifestyle. However, Rosann's comprehensive approach to health and the insight into gut and hormone health had me intrigued.

Rosann gave me the hard truth I needed to hear about sugar in a way that I finally accepted. She made me realize that not dealing properly with my excess stress was affecting me physiologically. She taught me about the nutrients I needed most in a way that I finally understood, including convincing me to eat avocados, which are not my favorite. She convinced me that despite everything else I have going on, my health had to be at the top of the list, a truth that I had been avoiding for a while.

Almost a year later, I've lost seventeen pounds. I have upped my fitness game to a level I couldn't even envision a year ago. My headaches are virtually gone and my stomach is calm. I am making real food, made with real ingredients, on a regular basis. My sugar consumption is down exponentially. I've found the right combination of vitamins and minerals to optimize my own personal health. I have learned to love weight lifting, challenging hikes, and long bike rides. In short, I feel like a badass.

I urge you to tap into your inner fire and apply it to your health and all aspects of life. Especially if you are a woman in your forties or beyond, you need to equip yourself to be in the driver's seat of your health. You have a choice. You can continue on autopilot and battle the inevitable health challenges that come with that path. Or you can learn about approaches to build a strong, lean, and healthy body and apply them. The choice is clear – and you are worth it.

This past year I have logged plenty of time on Rosann's couch for coaching sessions - learning, celebrating, game-planning, even shedding a few tears, receiving compassion and support for when life got crazy, and at times tough love and a push forward. Most recently I've been spending time in her home gym learning new workouts, laughing, and getting strong. Rosann has poured all of this insight into this book, creating a tool that, if you choose to take advantage of it, will change the trajectory of your health and your life.

Get the match ready; it is time to light that fire!

MOLLY MERCER
Chief Financial Officer, Slippery Rock University
Fellow Badass

Contents

Introduction

"And one day she discovered that she was fierce, strong, and full of fire, and that not even she could hold herself back because her passion burned brighter than her fears."

— MARK ANTHONY

If there were ever a statement more boldly true, it would be this one: Life is *fucking* hard! I'm confident that is a certainty we will both agree on. If you haven't experienced a single gut-wrenching hardship up to this point in your life, you must be an alien from another planet, or perhaps you've just been lucky enough to dodge a bullet a time or two. I suspect that isn't the case. Otherwise, you never would have curiously picked up this book in the first place.

We all struggle at some point. Call it disappointment, failure, heartbreak, tragedy, horrifying, or something else from a long list of other descriptive words that come up during the hardest times of our lives.

But, equip ourselves physically and mentally? We overcome! We conquer!

I assure you; this book is not going to be all doom and gloom. That's not who I am as a person, and indeed not the message I care to spread. It is essential to reflect on the hard things we face, because it's in the heat of the toughest moments in our lives where our character, fortitude, and strength unite. Hardships will always surface in life. What we do with them, determines everything in our future health and happiness.

I like to refer to this combination as the initial spark that, given the right elements, will become a burning hot wildfire within. That fire is not a bad thing! It lights up your life and sets you up to achieve your best self. In the end, it becomes your legacy!

"Health is not valued until sickness comes."
– THOMAS FULLER

I am thankful to have been blessed beyond measure in so many ways. While I admit I have truly lived a great and very fulfilling life, some may think everything is always perfect for me. I promise it's not. Even now, as I write this, I'm going through some shit. It happens. Sometimes, it happens a lot! I've been through various levels of hell the past 40+ years. I'm sure you can relate to some of it.

I know very personally how scary and heartbreaking it is as a 6-year-old when Mom and Dad get divorced and live in different states. I know what it's like to have money, and I know what it's like to live paycheck to paycheck - literally down to the last penny. I know the insecurities that grow when you're the social outcast in school. I understand the desperation and fear of living in an abusive relationship and the struggle to find your way out.

I know the frustration of working your ass off to climb that corporate ladder, only to be laid off years later. I know the over-whelm of being a stepmom, a first-time mom, a stay-at-home mom, and a mom to daughters. Don't get me wrong. Mother-hood? Without question, the greatest blessing and the best experience of my entire life! Also, the scariest. And most demand-ing.

I know how it feels to want more from life—like there's a higher purpose you have yet to achieve—and not know where, what, or how to figure it all out. I know what it's like to watch someone you love experience loss and depression and to feel so damn helpless to fix the problem. I know the pain of long-term unemployment, dwindled love, chronic stress, divorce, and the consequences of major life mistakes.

I know how heartbreaking it is to be judged for every choice and to lose friendships over it. I understand feelings of inadequacy. I know the pure hell of loving someone who doesn't love back. I know loneliness and struggle. I know what it's like to live more than 2200 miles away from any family members while going through the hardest season of my life. I know the heartache and grief of losing a parent unexpectedly.

I know, have lived with, and thoroughly understand regret.

I also know what it's like to lose my health and fight like hell to regain it. That is the cornerstone, the pivoting point in my life that led to a career as a health and wellness professional writing this book for you.

What the Hell Happened When I Turned 40?

They say the older we get, the more our body begins to fall apart. People talk about it like it's normal. Acceptable even. When you're young and healthy, the last thing you anticipate having happen is a failure in the mechanics of the well-designed, super machine that keeps you breathing, smiling, working, and playing.

Unfortunately, when we think we're invincible, we abuse the shit out of our body. We feed it processed foods, drink too much, smoke, abuse drugs, overload on energy drinks and caffeine, and load up on sugar like it's crack. We burn the candle at both ends, work insane hours, and joke about how we'll sleep when we're dead.

We're always staring at some screen, wondering why our life isn't as impressive as the Jones'. In our relationships, we blame him or her rather than taking personal responsibility, and we pick fights not worth pursuing.

We create a toxic environment both inside and outside of our body.

News flash—our body eventually breaks down. It's not that single sugar-coated Dunkin Donut, the grudge you refuse to release, or the one night you went out and drank yourself so silly you don't remember much of what happened that caused the breakdown. It's the cumulative effect of a lifetime of poor choices that overwhelm our body's ability to process all of it efficiently.

For me, that eye-opening event occurred when I turned 40.

It had admittedly been a solid 22 years of neglecting my body in one form or another and often in multiple ways that led to my breakdown. The thing is, I had no idea the choices I was making were causing so much internal stress, inflammation, or systemic imbalance. I was utterly clueless about my own human body. For most of my life, I believed, or had never really contemplated if it were possible, that I was invincible. Circumstances beyond my control that led to chronic stress were part of the problem. I lacked knowledge and understanding of the importance of nourishing my body through the tough times.

But there I was, 40 years old, feeling the mechanics of my body were failing. I felt different but couldn't put my finger on why or what exactly was wrong. I just knew something was off. I didn't feel right.

Foods that I usually had no trouble eating, I suddenly couldn't digest well. Gas, bloating, heartburn, indigestion, and irregular bowel movements were never an issue before, but now it was my daily reality.

My ability to fall asleep and stay asleep at night - gone! I had always been a great sleeper, but anxiety (one more thing I had never struggled with) was keeping me awake. I would feel my heart rate decrease and my breathing slow down so much that I'd start to panic, hyperventilate, and worry that closing my eyes would result in death while I was asleep.

Exercise recovery was suddenly horrible, leaving me feeling debilitated by massive fatigue and headaches. About an hour after my workout, I would have to lay down and sleep off the problem. If I tried to take Motrin for it, my stomach would feel a burning sensation, just one more thing that was out of the normal.

My weight started to leap upward despite all of my efforts to get thinner. It made no sense. I was burning more calories than I was consuming, yet I was gaining weight, and all in my mid-section! Everything within me questioned how that was even possible.

Energy was non-existent. My get-up-and-go got up and left, and I had no idea why or how to fix it. I struggled to be able to pull myself up off the couch long enough to do basic tasks around the house like loading the dishwasher or swapping out a load of laundry.

The unknown hormone imbalance I was dealing with caused me to feel moody as hell. I could see myself snapping emotionally at the stupidest things. I even booted friends out of my life like it was no big deal and felt a strange sense of relief from having done so. My whole family had to walk on eggshells around me for fear of saying or doing something that would set me off.

Probably one of the hardest nuts to swallow during all of this was hearing my then 8-year-old daughter ask on multiple occasions, "Mom, why can't we play together? Are you ever going to be healthy enough to play with me again?" Her words crushed my mama heart so much. I knew she didn't understand what was going on with me, and indeed, neither did I.

As I would try to navigate through each day, I'd feel shaky and nauseous. Sometimes I would wonder if I was pregnant, but that made no sense since I hadn't had a shred of libido for that to happen, and my menstrual cycle was strangely and suddenly quite the mess of irregularity.

Often, while attempting to relax and watch TV, I would suddenly feel like I was trembling from within. It was like my nervous system was about to jump right out of my skin. Everyone thought I was crazy, but I knew I wasn't. Something was wrong with my health!

These strange symptoms weighed heavy on me every day. I began to wonder if I was dying, which led to a full-blown anxiety attack one evening over dinner. It's not a regular occurrence to have all of your extremities entirely in a state of pins and needles. A trip to the emergency room finally revealed some answers.

At the hospital, they drew blood and discovered I had an electrolyte imbalance, so they gave me a potassium pill which almost immediately calmed my symptoms down. Then they diagnosed me with anxiety and told me to follow up with my doctor.

The following week, while sitting in my doctor's office, the physician's assistant told me that my blood work from the hospital indicated elevated TSH levels (thyroid-stimulating hormone) which would point to hypothyroidism, most likely Hashimoto's Disease. "If you're going to have a disease, thyroid disease is the easiest to treat," she said with a smile.

I was so thrilled to have answers and to know I wasn't going crazy. There *was* something wrong with me! What I didn't realize was that her statement was a damn lie. Thyroid disease is not at all easy to treat, and anyone who struggles with it would agree 100% with me on that. Within two weeks of my diagnosis, I had started and stopped taking thyroid medication, sought out a second opinion from a different doctor, and started the journey of restoring my health holistically.

My first instinct after my diagnosis had been to Google a variety of keywords and phrases related to Hypothyroidism, Hashimoto's, and Thyroiditis. That's something I don't recommend in any scenario of a health struggle. There are so many horror stories out there! Everyone's body and circumstances are entirely different, so your unique journey to healing will be much different than someone else's.

It took me two years to get my thyroid levels back to where they should have been all along. I had to become my own health advocate, research everything, try this or that, and read book after book on the subject of thyroid health, hormone balance, and aging. I even went as far as reading the literature concerning the hormonal birth control pills I had been taking.

Not gonna lie. Those two years sucked so bad! The thyroid affects every cell in your body so when there's not enough hormone circulating, or the hormone isn't able to be received by the cells, the symptoms one can experience are vast and frequently debilitating. What doesn't kill you certainly makes you stronger and more knowledgeable. That was my story.

I soaked up so much knowledge on my journey to healing, and

I am forever grateful that I had a reliable support system of family, friends, and even the most fantastic family medicine doctor who more or less let me tell *him* what I needed. I also had input from a few key people in the natural health field who helped me dig deep to treat the root cause of my health issues.

What I discovered through this process was that I felt immensely better when I removed certain foods from my diet, added others, drank more water, reduced sugar, and significantly modified my lifestyle choices, including a big focus on stress reduction. Unfortunately, there is no quick fix when we've let our body and our health be our lowest priority for so long. Consistency and dedication were critical factors in my success.

Transformed into Nutrition and Fitness Pro

It was at the point of healing that my first initial spark of passion around health, wellness, and nutrition began to heat up within me. My new purpose in life had suddenly surfaced. I felt strongly that I needed to learn more and use that knowledge to help others going through similar challenges in their health.

But first, life led me to a local martial arts academy where I developed a passion for MMA, specifically Kickboxing and Krav Maga, an Israeli self-defense fighting style. After a year of never missing a class, my instructor trained and certified me to teach Kickboxing, and he also taught me everything I now know as an advanced student in Krav Maga. I eventually broadened my horizons from fighting with my hands and feet to training to proficiency at the pistol range, which was all incredibly empowering and confidence-building. Meanwhile, my health continued to improve.

It wasn't long after I got my clean bill of health, that I enrolled for study with the Institute for Integrative Nutrition®, the world's largest nutrition school. One year later I launched my nutrition health coaching business, and I have gone on to receive training in hormone health and gut health, as well as a National Academy of Sports Medicine certification as a Personal Trainer.

For me, this journey wasn't just about improving my physical health, although initially, that was the primary focus. It was also about learning to find and control my inner fighting spirit, and then nourish my life in a multitude of ways that I hadn't before. All of this grew my confidence, inspired me to break free from what was holding me back, allowed me to find myself, and it fueled my inner fire to burn so fucking hot that people started to take notice.

There's no question in my mind - everything I had been through in my life up to this fourth decade, and all of the stress I allowed my body to endure, took a severe toll on my physical and mental health. My fire had nearly extinguished. But, thankfully, there was still just enough spark within me. All it needed was a little extra heat, quality fuel, and plenty of oxygen.

If I've learned anything the past twenty years, it's been that it's not the trial itself, but how we respond to it—that inner fire within us—that determines whether it makes us or breaks us. When we are burning hot from within, our potential to overcome obstacles and succeed in those big, hairy, audacious goals we set for ourselves is nearly out of this world. The choice to be a victim or a badass is yours.

What are you facing that has your stomach in knots? What health struggle is making you feel weak and overwhelmed? Are you sick and tired of feeling sick and tired? Do you hate what you see when you look in the mirror? Are you feeling trapped in your current situation? Is life feeling like nothing more than a boring rat race?

Well, then it's time for you to take bold, courageous, badass steps toward health, healing, and happiness. You get one shot at this life. That's it. It's short, it's fast, and it will require bold action. Don't think for one second you don't have what it takes to change things. You do!

Our effort becomes our reality. If you aren't happy with some aspect of your present situation, if you want to change your life, your health, and your happiness, it's going to take hard work. It's going to take dedication, time, commitment, an open mind, and a strong desire to achieve your fullest potential.

Let's face it. You're gonna have to become a badass.

There's no easy way to do it. No magic pill that makes the weight fall off or the health condition suddenly heal. There is no room for laziness or excuses. The truth is, if you aren't willing to sweat a little, to get creative with your time, to try new foods, or to be open-minded to solutions that all point to a better you and a better life, then this book is NOT for you, and neither is the health coaching you would otherwise get from me.

I know that may sound harsh, and I don't like excluding people from an opportunity to transform their life completely. But I've been working as an Integrative Nutrition Health Coach and Personal Trainer long enough to know that a person who doesn't have skin in the game or who isn't willing to change will not be successful in their attempts, no matter how much guidance I offer or how much I work with them on developing new habits and shifting their mindset.

It goes back to the question, "how bad do you want it?" When you really want something, it happens. When it's not essential to you, excuses happen.

Odds are, you already know what you need to do to be healthier, you just don't know where to start or how to keep going. You don't know how to resist temptations or avoid self-sabotage. You don't have support from someone who genuinely cares about your success. If you did, you never would have picked up this book and started reading it. What you need is that kick-in-the-ass accountability from a professional.

That's where I get to do what I love so much! Every day I'm privileged to help my clients discover their unique inner spark, and then I teach them how to add fuel, increase the heat, and supply that flame with oxygen, so it grows into a wild blaze of passion. Another way of inspiring change is that I hold their feet to the fire the entire time! Accountability can be a real bitch, but it is effective in most cases.

In my mind, it's a job well done when I can watch a quiet, re-served mom of two, lacking confidence in her abilities, and aching for order and direction in her life, come out of my coaching program twenty pounds lighter, glowing with joy, and as a brand new badass entrepreneur.

That's just one example of a real-life win I've been privileged to be a part of as I've grown this nutrition and fitness coaching practice of mine. That beautiful client is now a lovely friend, and she had a spark that grew into a blaze of passion and continues to grow!

Not only have I been blessed to be able to work with clients helping them find the health and happiness they deserve, but I've practiced what I know and preach in my own life and have com-pletely transformed my energy levels, my creativity, my confidence, my relationships, my understanding of the body, and well... my level of badassery, too!

If I could work in a coach/client relationship with every person who picks up this book, I would! But there is only one of me and not nearly enough hours in a week. So, this book is my way of getting my message - my health coaching - out to the world, at least on some beginner level.

It's worth repeating. Life is *fucking* hard. But I don't believe in letting hardships destroy me or sit there in my mind as this horrible memory. I think somehow using our pain to create healing and hope for others is wise. I choose to be that woman who, despite going through hell, emerges from the flames carrying buckets of water for anyone else who may need help.

It is, without a doubt, my greatest passion as a health and well-ness professional to help inspire positive change in the lives of those who know me and work with me. I love watching people dig deep, suck it up, walk it off, work hard, and stay committed to the cause all to become their best self. I love watching health and happiness bloom!

In the pages that follow, I'll be walking you through the fire triangle as it relates to life nourishment, body nourishment, and physical strength and vitality. You'll discover the secrets I live in my own life and teach to my clients for their healthiest lives. Some things I share may be new information you've never heard, and others may be a fresh perspective on something you've known all along but have failed to perfect for yourself.

I'm genuinely excited to share this knowledge and my thoughts with you, as this book has been brewing in me for many years. But, as is the case with most things in life, timing is everything.

I hope that this is your time! Your time to finally have answers, feel hope again, and experience success in making your life and your health everything you've always wanted it to be. You certainly deserve to thrive!

I believe there's a flame inside of you right this moment. Let's make it burn hot, shall we?

PART 1

Creating Inner Fire

How Your Inner Fire Fuels a Healthy Life

"Everything you need to be great is already inside of you. Stop waiting for someone or something to light your fire. You have the match."

– UNKNOWN

Fire has always been somewhat fascinating to me. Depending on the circumstances, that flicker of orange can be stunning, or it can be wildly unpredictable. Throughout my life, I've had many experiences with fire, but seeing what a wildfire looks like at night is one image I'll never forget.

My mom and I, with friends, were stopped in bumper to bumper traffic on a single lane road somewhere between Idaho and Northern California. The night sky should have been black and starry. Instead, all I could see was a bright red glow! Looking out the backseat window, I could see flames in the brush along the side of the road. Through my 9-year-old eyes, I would swear it was like an angry 15-foot tall, endlessly vast beast coming right at us. Paralyzed in fear, I could only stare out the window at the monstrosity of that fire.

I don't recall most of the details of our drive that evening, but I'm still alive to tell some of the story, so it must not have been as bad as I thought it was. Although that *was* the night, I developed a newfound respect for the power of fire. Since then, I've contemplated our own inner fire, and the questions, "why do we call it inner fire and what creates it in each of us?" I now have my own theory on how to compare the magnitude and the beauty of physical fire with that of our own deepest passions and inner fire.

Whether it's burning up a hillside near your neighborhood or burning hot within your soul, fire can most definitely be a scary thing! In both scenarios, it has the potential to be extremely dangerous, destructive, and even unpredictable. But fire can also be beneficial. It can be, in most cases, precisely what we need! I know, crazy, but stick with me here.

Fire, in and of itself, is not bad most of the time. It's quite useful in improving our quality of life. Think about it - fire lights the way, keeps us warm, and inspires passion. It roasts our marshmallows, boils water, and is sterilizing. When we're in a bind, fire signals for rescue, and it repels bugs. You must add "see fire dancing" to your bucket list if you haven't already seen it. Fire can be very entertaining! And let's not dismiss the fact that a wildfire leaves our ecosystem well-nourished. One more exciting thing to note: The Bible tells us that fire represents God's radiant glory as an aspect of His Holiness (Heb 12:29).

Fire is not a thing, but rather an event. Without fuel, heat, and oxygen, it cannot ever take place. Those are the three elements necessary for the chemical reaction, or spontaneous combustion, resulting in the creation of a physical fire.

Our inner fire, responsible for bringing our strong-minded, success-driven, intelligent, confident, energetic, highly competitive, fearless, badass-self out for the world to see, is also an event.

You may not know that DNA fluoresces. Yes, that's right. It emits light without outside help. We literally are beings of light! And that fire is created and grows in much the same way, and even with the same magnitude, as a physical fire. The goal is to fuel our bodies adequately, then add heat and oxygen. This raises your frequency or energy – the rate at which your body, your cells, vibrate, and it will cause your fire to burn unmistakably hot, sometimes even to the point of being a little bit wild. If you remove or reduce any of the elements mentioned, your inner fire will die down to nothing more than a smoldering. When it dies completely, your physical life ends.

Just like a physical fire, caution is always necessary when keeping our inner fire regulated. A well-nurtured, controlled fire can ignite passion, ambition, creativity, strength, and courage. These are all healthy qualities to have. Let the flame burn too out of control, and we risk becoming reckless or even quick to anger. Let one or more elements of the fire triangle slide, and the result is a loss of enthusiasm, effort, and determination. This equates to life-sucking things like laziness, lack of joy, nutritional deficiencies, obesity, stagnation, and eventually, chronic illness.

What is the current state of your inner fire? Are you feeling a low smolder? If so, keep reading. My goal is to fill your toolbox full of knowledge around what's healthy and what isn't, and then give you the kick-in-the-ass you need to stop making excuses, stop giving up on yourself, and stop doubting your ability to change. Your health and your life matter.

To be your best self, you have to stop saying you'll do it tomorrow, next week, next month, at the start of the new year, when life calms down, blah, blah, blah. Either you want it, or you don't. Today... right this moment... is the perfect time to chase the life and the dreams you desire!

SECRET #2

Believe in Yourself

"**I** can, and I will."

Those words must be a piece of the puzzle that is my genetic makeup. I believe in myself, even if I'm about to attempt something I've never done before. As long as I can remember, I have never backed down from a challenge, a fight, a goal, or anything I've set my heart's desire on conquering. Once I'm in, I'm all in, and I don't stop until victory is achieved.

I even joke with my clients that if I were to personally participate in my own Better Body Challenge© with them, knowing there was a monetary prize for the person with the greatest percentage of weight loss, I would win. Every time. No questions asked. It's not to say they couldn't possibly go head to head with me and beat me. I have no doubt many of them could! That's why I like to joke about it. Most are just as competitive as I am.

My confidence is rooted in knowing myself and my own strong-willed nature. I am way too determined, stubborn, competitive, free-spirited, ambitious, and way too on fire for this life of mine for there to be any other result that isn't a win. But all that inner drive and desire has to be fueled by something – and that fuel is my health! Not just "okay" health but outstanding health!

Without a healthy body, properly balanced hormones, a thriving gut and microbiome, and an optimally functioning brain, my vitality and joy for life diminishes! I've been down that path before, and I will never let myself go there again. Keeping my fire burning hot is the secret to living the quality of life I desire.

Maybe you're feeling depleted of your fuel. You want more confidence and to feel good in your body again. Perhaps you have no energy left for anything. You're feeling defeated and hopeless. Maybe your weight won't drop, or your digestive system is a mess. Perhaps your periods are irregular, or your hair is falling out. Your libido is non-existent. Maybe... fill-in-the-blank. The list could go on and on, but the bottom line is this: to overcome any of it, you first have to believe in yourself and know in your heart that you are capable of greatness. No matter how hard it will be to make changes, you've got this!

SECRET #3

Decide What You Want and

Be Fearless About It

You are a miracle. Do you realize the magnitude of that statement? Think about it. How many females do you think your dad crossed paths with in his life leading up to the day he met and sparked an interest in your mom? I'm gonna throw an estimate out there. Let's say 10,000 females. I know it seems like a high number, but it's probably not too far off.

Think about all the girls he went to high school and college with. What about the female co-workers he had? Did he ever travel for work before he met your mother? If so, there are thousands of women he could have crossed paths with in airports, hotel lobbies, and bars. It doesn't mean he talked with them or had a relationship with them. Just that the potential was there.

Same scenario for your mother. She was no doubt exposed to countless males throughout her high school, college, work, and traveling years. Yet somehow, one man and one woman – with the necessary pieces of your unique genetic makeup – met, had a conversation and decided from there to go on a date. There was chemistry between them on that date which miraculously led to a relationship that lasted long enough to fall in love, get married, and produce offspring.

If your dad had met, fallen in love with, and married some other woman, you wouldn't be here today. If your parents hadn't decided to go on that date with one another, you wouldn't be here today.

But let's dig a little deeper still.

You are the result of one single sperm and one single egg fusing together and creating your unique genetic makeup. The average woman has about 100,000 eggs that are released during her fertile years. A man produces about 12 trillion sperm during his reproductive years. The probability of that one egg and that one sperm coming together to create another human life is about one in 400 quadrillion.

It doesn't stop there, though. We still have to consider that 50% of all pregnancies end in miscarriage. Also, your ancestors had to experience this miracle of life themselves, meet up with the right male or female, survive the many risks in this world long enough to reproduce, and this scenario went on and on for generations until you arrived.

So you see, you are a miracle. You are here for a particular reason. You only have one life, and it's short. Here and gone in a breath. If you're drifting through life aimlessly, you will at some point reach the end of it with regrets, having never known or accomplished your full potential or your heart's greatest desire. Wouldn't you rather live life with passion and purpose? I know you would, because that is an almost ingrained piece of our humanity.

You may be wondering at this point what this all has to do with your health. Quite frankly, it has everything to do with your health. I'll be guiding you through what foods you should be eating for optimal health and vitality, but you need to understand that it's not just the food on your plate that determines how healthy you are as an individual.

In fact, a more significant determining factor in health starts in your gut, and chronic stress is detrimental to gut health. So, if you are experiencing any disappointment or lack of satisfaction in your life right now, it is negatively impacting your health. Not just your gut health, but also your immune system, your brain, your hormones, your digestive system, and your metabolism.

The first question I ask my clients is, "What do you want for yourself?" To answer that, a few other high mileage questions come into play, starting with addressing the real, bottom-line reason why we often don't do what's important to us.

It's an ugly word, and it's called fear.

I don't know about you, but I believe it would be a damn shame to reach the end of your life filled with regret for not taking bold and courageous action towards the things you feel drawn to. One thing I've learned the past few years is that a bold decision, while not always popular, can open doors and bring happiness you never thought possible. There is nothing wrong with stepping outside of your comfort zone. It's on the outskirts of what's most comfortable that our most considerable growth happens.

To illustrate the power of fear, I can tell you the story of elk in Yellowstone Park during the winter months. Food is scarce and temperatures can drop below zero, cold even for an elk. So they tend to huddle near the geysers where the hot mist keeps them warm. But many end up starving because there's no vegetation around the hot geyser. The few who are brave enough to wander just a hundred feet away find vegetation. It's the sweet spot between the too-hot geyser and the freezing cold. They survive because they left the comfort zone, while the others literally died from their fear.

So in order to decide what you want, we need to first address fear.

What would you do if you weren't afraid? It is a fantastic question, and one worth taking the time to really reflect on. Asking yourself that simple, yet tough question could lead to uncovering your deepest desires, why they matter so much, and why you haven't yet achieved them.

Inside of you are specific gifts and talents that help to give you a sense of purpose and passion. Be it a knack for crocheting, a beautiful singing voice, a love for educating children, a heart for supporting victims of sex-trafficking, or your own heartbreaking story that can be used to love and help others in their journey, you have something of value to offer this world.

22

It's said that if you love what you do, you'll never work a day in your life. I believe that to be true. It certainly has been for me as I've been running my own health and fitness business. I literally wake up excited to do the work that I do! I get to inspire change in the lives of my clients, encourage them, educate them, and push them to meet the goals that will ultimately help them to be their best self.

When you're passionate about something, nothing stands in your way. You're all in. Your mind runs nonstop thinking of fresh new ideas and techniques you can develop and implement to continue growing in your passion. I can't tell you how many nights I've woken up at 2am with busy-brain. I'll have some business growth idea hit me and my brain will decide to map it all out in the middle of the night. Innovation and persistence is the life of an entrepreneur. It's exciting and it's what I love!

Life is too short to be dull. You shouldn't feel bored or unfulfilled, and you definitely shouldn't be okay with just being mediocre. Find your passion. Know your purpose. Let it light you up like nothing else ever has.

Nelson Mandela said, "There is no passion to be found in playing small—in settling for a life that is less than the one you are capable of living." If I could high-five him for that statement, I would. I couldn't agree more! Take a look at the work and the hobbies you currently do. Are they consuming you? Do you wake up excited to tackle another day and another project? Are you going to sleep at night still thinking about it? If you can't honestly say yes to those questions, you need to start doing some soul searching. One life. That's all you have. Make it count!

If you aren't sure what your purpose or passions are, it's okay. It doesn't have to be anything fancy or wild. You get to decide for yourself what lights your fire. Odds are, it's right there hanging out in the forefront of your mind. You can reflect on some high-mileage questions and do some journaling around your answers to explore this more.

- What are you super curious about?
- What do you do really well that others are frequently complimenting you for?
- What do people seek out your expertise or opinion on?
- What hobbies or talents have you pursued throughout your life and why?
- If money wasn't an issue, what would you do with your time?
- What do you love to do?
- What do you feel called to do?

It may take some hard experiences and a little self-reflection to discover precisely what it is you are meant to be doing and what will bring you the most joy and satisfaction in this life. Maybe there's someone you watch from afar that is always on some mission to improve the world or him- herself. Keep watching, and let that person inspire fresh ideas for your own future.

Be careful not to let your insecurities get in the way. The negative thoughts going through your head are not your reality unless you allow them to be. I call these the thought police, constantly trying to regulate your thoughts so you don't think outside the box. It might be an excellent time for you to step outside of your day to day norm and do something you've never done before. That's how I developed a passion for mixed martial arts. I had never done anything quite like a martial arts form of kickboxing or Krav Maga. But as soon as I started, I was hooked! One thing led to another and now that is a part of my mindset and it's integrated into my coaching practice. Had I never stepped foot in that martial arts academy, I wouldn't have the desire, the skill, or the knowledge of self-defense that I have today.

What would make your life shine brighter and feel more meaningful? Most of the time, areas of dissatisfaction are a result of that crazy emotion called fear. You may be thinking you have valid reasons for being in the particular situation you're in, and you're probably right. But I encourage you to take some time to peel back the layers.

If you do, I'd be willing to bet you'd uncover the true culprit – you're afraid.

It's okay to be afraid, as long as you don't let it stall you out on living the life you want. Sometimes fear is a good thing, alerting you and protecting you from potentially harmful situations. Beware, though, fear can be destructive to your soul, to your health, and to your happiness if your fears are not justified by some actual fearful event.

Most of the time, unreasoning fear is the result of some past event that you perceived as negative. So now you have what's called catastrophic thinking. You think any situation that resembles that past negative experience is going to turn out the same way. I hate to say this, but it's all in your head. Literally.

If you've been feeling paralyzed and stuck on an issue, or you feel unable to move forward with or make some necessary changes in your life, that is a sign of the not-so-good fear creeping in. Bad fear will literally stop you in your tracks and hold you back from fully experiencing life. Your confidence will suffer, and as a result, you'll avoid taking any kind of courageous action. Fear will ultimately prevent you from growing as an individual, and your life will become stagnant.

So I ask again…

What would you do if you weren't afraid?

Think about it.

- *Would you jump out of an airplane?*
- *Would you go Facebook Live and tell everyone watching what you are most passionate about in this whole world?*
- *Would you quit your job?*
- *Would you start your own business?*
- *Would you sign up for boxing lessons?*
- *Would you make a commitment to your health and stick with it for the long haul?*

In my 46 years, I've learned a whole lot of life lessons, but the past few years has probably been my most exceptional period of personal growth and development.

Why?

Because every decision I've made has been one of action, despite how scared to death I was of taking those steps. I'm talking about bold, courageous, knee-shaking action! It's been good for me, though, and I assure you it will be equally great for you!

Taking bold action has allowed me to experience both wins and losses that have looked like this:

- success
- weight loss
- personal growth
- new knowledge
- new love
- great disappointment
- broken relationships
- enormous stress
- incredible freedom
- soaring confidence
- business growth
- revived independence
- and... hope.

One of the best quotes I've heard and have come to live by is by Joshua Rosenthal, founder of the Institute for Integrative Nutrition®. Joshua always says, "Feel the fear and do it anyway." I love that because it always results in positive growth.

Failure is always success. Either you succeed or you learn. There is no failure. I want to challenge you to stop living your life on autopilot. Instead, acknowledge your obstacles and jump forward despite how scary they appear. If you aren't happy or something about your situation is putting out your inner fire, *do something about it.* Take bold action and change your circumstances. You hold power to do so, even if you think you don't. Kick the excuses to the curb and take control of things.

Make a commitment to your health. Lose those unwanted pounds. Speak up about what's bothering you. End that toxic relationship. Take the leap to go back to school. Pay attention to what sucks the life and joy out of you and change it! Take action. At some point, you have to stop thinking about it, planning out every scenario, and just freaking go for it. Don't just stand on the edge of the diving board. If you want to swim, you have to jump in.

You can start all of this by giving your fears a shape. Think about how exactly they have power over you and why. What do they look like? Are they even realistic? What is triggering those fearful thoughts in the first place? How are your fears preventing you from enjoying excellent health and the life you've always wanted?

It helps to visualize your dream life, too. What is it that you really want? Take some time today to block out all of the noise and really imagine in your mind's eye what your dream life would look like, feel like, and yes, even what it would taste like! Jot down a list of as many things as you can think of that you would do in a heartbeat if you weren't afraid of the possible consequences. Remember that most of our fears are irrational, meaning the worst-case scenario we are creating in our minds would never actually happen.

Once you have a clear picture in your mind of what you want to experience or achieve in your life, the next step is to break it down into mini-goals that you can work on. This makes getting there feel less overwhelming while also giving you opportunities to succeed and celebrate along the way. Also, your confidence will grow, which will build momentum in your stride and help you to keep going. One crucial point, though – don't hesitate to first confront the areas of your life that are most out of alignment with your desires! Out with the bad, in with the awesome!

Every time you overcome a significant obstacle, take time to celebrate the fact that you are no longer living in fear. Be proud that you are conquering anything that gets in the way of your happiness!

SECRET #4

Know your Why

Once you've decided what you want and you're feeling pretty badass and fearless about it, the next step is to know why it matters to you. Knowing your "why" will keep you motivated to continue the journey, even on those days when you just don't feel like taking the time to throw together a healthy lunch – Wendy's drive-thru just seems so much easier, right?

Usually, our why is tied to an emotional trigger. Maybe you were picked on in school for being overweight, and it's a constant battle with your self-confidence. Or perhaps you've experienced or have watched someone you love go through a health problem resulting from poor diet and lifestyle choices.

I shared in the introduction of this book how I landed in this health and wellness career. It all began with a wrong diagnosis of Hashimoto's Thyroiditis. The way I felt while going through that health struggle was the worst I've ever felt in my life. It was literally debilitating physically, emotionally, and mentally. It took me a long time to figure out how to heal my body and get back to optimal health.

Because of that experience, I will never let myself get sick like that again. It is my personal emotional trigger.

When I think about that tough season of life, to this day, I still get choked up over it. It was *that* hard! I've never valued my health more than I do now.

Having recently gone through a marital separation and divorce, while also mourning the sudden death of my mother, the past year has been one of high emotional stress. I know how my body responds to the emotional stress of that nature, and how easily it can slip back into a thyroid or other hormone imbalance as a result.

To be proactive in my health and happiness, I've had to be very intentional about remembering my why, keeping my nutrition on point, getting enough sleep, exercising regularly, supporting my body with stress-management supplementation, and taking time to play and socialize with family and friends.

So you see, we all have an emotional trigger that points our heart in the direction of what is truly best for us. Not only do you have to *want* to be healthier, but you need to know *why* it matters. You also need to be willing to make hard decisions that position you and your life for what you want out of it regardless of what naysayers may say.

Your why can be a powerful motivator in helping you make the hard choices you know you need to make. What's your emotional trigger? What brings tears to your eyes when you think about this journey of getting healthier? Take some time right now to contemplate these questions and your answers.

My favorite and most compelling question for you to consider is this one:

If you don't change your current behaviors, choices, or situation, what will it cost you in the long run? What will it cost your loved ones?

The emotional trigger is your why. If there's no emotion behind it, it will never be sufficient enough to keep you pointed in the right direction, focused on achieving your goal, or staying the course when the going gets tough — and it will get tough!

SECRET #5

Create a Vision Board

I suggest you take some time to create your own vision board to help bring your desires front and center. A vision board is an awesome tool used to help define, meditate, and maintain focus on specific life goals.

On your vision board will be images and phrases that reflect the life you want to live, the body you want to see when you look in the mirror, the health you want to experience, and the joy that will come from achieving all of these goals.

You can also display images of what you *don't* desire as a very visual reminder of the consequences that will occur from losing focus or falling off the wagon, so to speak. I also suggest writing your own personal mission statement and adding that to your vision board as well.

MISSION STATEMENT TEMPLATE
To [what you want to do] by [how you'll do it] so that [what result you hope to have.]

SAMPLE MISSION STATEMENT
To <u>fuel my fire</u> **by** <u>implementing life nourishment, body nourishment, and physical strength and vitality habits</u>, **so that** <u>I can live my healthiest and most fulfilling life</u>.

Your vision board can be created digitally, which I prefer because you can literally take it anywhere with you as long as you have your device on hand, or you can create one out of poster board and magazine or newspaper clippings. There are some great apps you can try out for a digital vision board. Look into *Corkulous, Dream Vision Board, Jack Canfield Vision Board by Mogulworx, Hay House Vision Board*, and *Dream Cloud* to see what works best for you and your personal preference.

SECRET #6

Set Health and Happiness Goals

Now that you know what you want out of life and why it matters, it's time to set your goals and begin to take action. Keep in mind a goal without a plan is just a wish, so let's work on evaluating areas of weakness in your life, setting your goals, and creating a plan to bring your desires to fruition.

Life Evaluation Chart

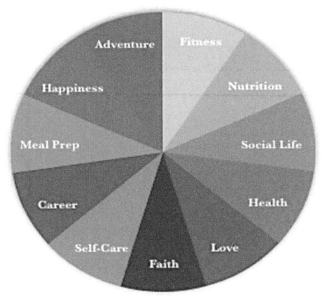

Start by evaluating the different categories in the Life Evaluation Chart above. For each category ask yourself this question, "How satisfied am I in this area of life?" Then give it a rating on a scale from 1 to 10. [1 = needs serious improvement, 10 = doing great.]

Once you've determined which areas of life need the most attention, pick 3 to start tackling immediately. Come up with a specific goal for each one that will greatly improve your rating in those categories. Next, break those goals down into smaller ones that are S.M.A.R.T. (specific, measurable, active, realistic, and time bound.) Then give yourself a deadline for each one.

Let's say you weigh 150 pounds and you'd like to lose 30 pounds and tone up your body in time for bikini season. If bikini season is only 4 weeks away, losing 30 pounds is not realistic or a safe pace for weight loss. This doesn't mean you throw in the towel and do nothing. It means you start somewhere and begin to make progress. A safe pace is about 1-2 pounds per week. So, your goals could look like this instead.

On the surface, I realize this seems very repetitive. Why not just set one big goal to lose 30 pounds in 15 weeks? My answer to that is because you will have greater success if you break it down into smaller goals that are less overwhelming, that are healthy and sustainable, and that are reasonably easy to achieve. When you see success, the momentum to keep going will continue.

Really take the time to think about how you write out your goals because if you say, "I want to be healthier in 4 weeks," how in the world will you measure that to see if you actually are healthier?

Here's a breakdown explaining a little bit more what S.M.A.R.T goals look like:

(S) – Specific. A goal should be clearly defined, using details to describe specifically what the goal will be. So it's not enough to say "I want to lose weight." You must specify exactly how many pounds you want to lose. "I want to lose fifteen pounds."

(M) – Measurable. You must be able to measure a clear beginning and ending to your goal, with measurable results. "I now weigh 165 pounds. In thirty days I will weigh 150 pounds."

(A) – Active. You must take active responsibility for achieving the goal.

Passive: "I'm going to lose fifteen pounds if I ever get enough time to go to the gym." This puts no responsibility on you.

Active: "I'm going to lose fifteen pounds by the end of January."

(R) – Realistic. Any goal you set must be realistic. "I'm going to lose one hundred pounds in thirty days" is not only unrealistic, it's dangerous, but losing fifteen pounds in thirty days is very realistic and doable with the proper tools and actions.

(T) – Time Bound. Every goal must have a timeframe within which it will be completed. Businesses don't reach goals by saying to their employees "Here's a project for you, but it really doesn't matter when you get it done." When will you have those fifteen pounds off, exactly?

Having your S.M.A.R.T. plan in writing will keep you organized and allow you to see where you are in the process rather than trying to remember what you have to do and when.

One final thought about setting goals is this: Accountability! You are more likely to achieve the goals you've set for yourself when you tell people what you're doing and give them updates. So tell the world what you're up to.

Why Most People Fail to Achieve Their Goals

Many of the following excuses are reasons people fall short of achieving their goals. They're common excuses, so I'd be willing to bet you have had one or more come out of your mouth a time or two. I know I certainly have! Going forward, be very aware of these excuses. It's really important that you challenge yourself to press beyond them and live your life to the fullest. You will never regret shifting your mindset.

Excuse #1: *I don't have time.*

It's not really that you don't have time, you simply haven't chosen to make your health and happiness a priority. We all have the same 24 hours in a day. We make time for things that are important to us.

Excuse #2: *I don't have the knowledge.*

Well, reading this book is a significant first step! However, you may feel too overwhelmed by change, and so you close your mind to it completely. You may find working one-on-one with me as your health coach brings more notable success.

Excuse #3: *I don't like commitment.*

You can't say you want to lose weight and get healthier, stop at McDonald's on the way home from work and then park yourself in front of the TV the rest of the night. When it comes to achieving a healthier body and life, you need to give it 100% commitment and take 100% action towards making it happen.

Excuse #4: *It's too hard. I give up!*

The Better Body Challenge© is a 6-week online group nutrition and fitness coaching program I offer, but by the halfway point, many of my clients start to slack off and, in some cases, give up.

Getting healthy and making changes to your life takes time. It takes consistent effort every day! Don't give up the first time you don't see results. You're better than that! Extraordinary people go through many setbacks, failures, challenges, and hardships and never give up! Eventually, your persistence will pay off.

Excuse #5: *I'm just not feeling it right now.*

Taking action means stepping outside your comfort zone – trying new foods, new ways of cooking, new ways of moving your body, and new ways of coping with the stress of life. Choose to live each day with self-discipline, with your principles leading the way, not your feelings.

Excuse #6: *I'm afraid to fail.*
Failure is inevitable from time to time. Instead of worrying about it, shift your mindset. Either you'll win or you'll learn. Thomas Edison failed more than 10,000 times, but he never looked at his attempts as failures. Instead, he said that he successfully found 10,000 ways that didn't work. The only way you will fail is if you quit.

Excuse #7: *I'd rather do my own thing then follow this plan.*
In this book, I'll be teaching you the proper way to adequately nourish your body so you will feel amazing, and so that your body and all of your organs will function optimally. Derailing from this plan to "do your own thing" is your choice, but don't be upset with me if you don't get the results you were hoping for.

Excuse #8: *Everyone tells me it's a stupid idea.*
There will always be someone who tries to bring you down when you're making moves to improve yourself or your life. Don't listen to them. It's just their opinion and not your reality. The only limits you have are the limits you place on yourself. Nobody else gets to determine your success or your failure.

Excuse #9: *It's not working.*
Doubt comes into play when action is being taken but no results are happening. Or the results are happening very slowly. Trust the process! You didn't get to this particular place, weight, or health situation in your life overnight and you will not change your circumstances overnight either. Believe in yourself! You can do this!

Excuse #10: *Nobody else in my life is doing anything like this.*
You are the average of the 5 people you spend the most time with. Make sure you are spending time with people who aren't afraid to work hard, dream big, and push you toward success. Seek out a community of fellow healthy go-getters and strive for the same thing in your own life.

SECRET #7

Make a Commitment to Yourself

and Your Health

Commitment involves a strong desire to change and an action plan to do so. Consider this book your action plan. You'll find action steps throughout. I encourage you to take time to apply them in your own life. You've no doubt heard the saying, "You can lead a horse to water, but you can't make it drink." That same concept applies here. I will give you the tools, but if you don't implement them and use them consistently, you will not see the results you're capable of achieving.

So make a commitment to yourself and your health today. Shout it out to the world that you're reading this book and that you're taking steps to improve your life. When you share your level of commitment with others, you will be more likely to achieve the desires of your heart because there's added accountability in knowing people are watching you!

Those who know me personally and follow me on Facebook have watched my journey unfold over time. Every enormous goal I've set for myself, I've announced publicly on Facebook for the whole world to see, including the writing of this book. Scary? Hell, yes! But it has been instrumental in making sure I knock that goal out of the park because the last thing I want is for someone to be able to say, "I knew she couldn't do it."

Secrets to Making Your Health and Yourself a Priority

Take it in baby steps. Even if all you do is increase the amount of water you're drinking, you'll feel better, you'll create a new healthy habit, and you'll be motivated and energized to add another new healthy habit to your routine.

Change your attitude. It's much easier to stick with healthy change when we are excited about the changes we are about to make. Sometimes this means viewing exercise or healthy food through a different lens. For example, finding a way of exercising that lights your fire will shift your attitude from, "I have to exercise," to "I get to exercise!"

Get rid of the things that will derail you. If your kitchen is packed with junk food that you love and will be too much temptation, well… throw it all out. Instead, stock up with healthy snacks, get your hands on some great recipes, and purchase the necessary kitchen tools that will set you up for success. A great chef's knife goes a long way in making veggie chopping fun and easy!

Celebrate along the way. Small changes add up to significant results! Resist the temptation to compare your progress with someone else's. You are two very unique people with very individual circumstances. Eyes forward, chin up! Stay committed. Celebrate your victories. Recognize this truth: some of your wins may have nothing to do with the number on the scale.

Practice the 90/10 rule guilt-free. Everyone slips up from time to time. It's totally okay!! I believe in the 90/10 rule. This rule allows for a little bit of splurging so long as we are staying on point with nutrition and fitness the other 90% of the time. If you fall off track beyond that, don't stress about it. Just fix things with the very next choice you make.

Schedule your healthy habits like an appointment. Want to know how I get to the gym every day? How I walk my dog every day? How I drink enough water every day? How I enjoy self-care? I schedule or block it ruthlessly on my calendar and nothing, not even my kids, gets in the way of the appointment that is dedicated to my health and happiness.

If you're going to improve your life and get healthy, you need to make time for the action steps that are necessary, such as exercise, meal planning, home cooking, self-care, and sleep.

As we head forward into adding fuel to your inner fire, stay focused on the outcome rather than the obstacles. It won't be a comfortable journey, but it will be one that you'll never regret taking. Learning to fuel your fire and consistently provide it with what it needs to thrive is critical to having the health, the body, the life, and the happiness you desire!

Let's kickstart your fire now by taking action!

Fuel Your Fire Acton Steps:

1. Get clear on the current state of your inner fire.
2. Believe in yourself. You are more capable than you realize.
3. Decide what you want and be fearless about it.
4. Know your why, write it down, and put it in multiple places where you'll see it.
5. Create a vision board.
6. Write your personal mission statement. Put it on your vision board.
7. Set health and happiness goals.
8. Make a commitment to yourself and your health.

"Rosann has taught me how to find my highest self through the whirlwind of motherhood! My mind, body and spirit have reached goals that I didn't even know were possible. Thanks to her I have learned to use wellness and strength to become the strong badass woman that I am today!!"

– SARA BUZARD

PART 2

Add Nutrient-Dense Fuel
to Your Body

SECRET #8

Your Healthiest Life Begins with Water

"There's plenty of water in the universe without life, but nowhere is there life without water."

– SYLIVA A. EARLE

How much water have you had to drink today? It's a health coach accountability question I'm known for asking on a regular basis. They are words that make my clients cringe, because all too often, we aren't intentional enough about hydrating our bodies. And yet, it is a critical piece of the fuel that is a necessary element to creating your inner fire.

Water is essential for the human body to survive. You can go about three weeks without eating any food at all, but only three days without water. Every living cell in your body needs water to keep it functioning. You are literally made up of water (and bacteria). It is a major component of your blood, heart, lungs, brain, and bones.

Water is responsible for so many important tasks within your body. It helps your body to maintain the right temperature, it removes waste, and it also lubricates your joints. Additionally, water helps you digest your food through saliva and gastric secretions and nourishes your brain and spinal cord.

Here's what you may not realize. Even though your body is made up of water, you do still need to drink it because the rate you lose that water is pretty fast. Every day you are losing an average of

2 to 3 liters of water from sweating, breathing, urinating, and moving your bowels. That measurement increases if you are extremely active with exercise or sports. So taking in water and electrolytes daily from food and drinks is vital to maintaining electrolyte balance and proper hydration.

When I was pregnant, dehydration caused false labor. The hospital staff sent me home both times with strict instructions to drink more water. Years later, I began training hard at the gym and was drinking a ton of water. What I didn't know was that the hard level of training I was doing, coupled with years of chronic stress leading up to that point, negatively affected my adrenal health. My adrenals were pretty burned out and couldn't handle the workload of maintaining fluid and mineral balance in my body. Then one day, my arms, legs, fingers, and toes all went to sleep at the same time. It felt like a bad case of pins and needles all over. Talk about a scary feeling! It was an electrolyte imbalance. One potassium pill later, I felt like a completely different person.

While it is very individual, the average human body consists of 60-75% water. About 80% of brain tissue is made of water. Just a 2% reduction of water levels in the body can lead to a 20% decrease in mental and physical performance. Staying adequately hydrated has a critical impact on bodily functions like heart rate, blood pressure, muscle performance, and cognition.

If all you do differently today than you did yesterday is drink more water, you're already on the road to a healthier body. Most people don't drink enough water, though, and while water needs vary from person to person, it's actually one of the best things you can do to improve your health.

Age, sex, diet, activity level, and climate are all factors to be considered when determining how much water you should drink. If you're pregnant or have other health conditions, like kidney problems, for example, you should consult with your doctor for guidance.

For the average reasonably healthy person, it is generally suggested that you strive to drink at least half of your body weight in ounces of water per day. So, for example, a 150-pound individual would need to consume at least 75 ounces of water each day. Listen to your body and drink until you feel amazing.

Getting enough water during the day can often be a challenge for many. Start by purchasing a tumbler or water bottle you love. Depending on the size, maybe buy two or three of them. Fill them all up with water and put them in the fridge. As you go through your day, pull one from the fridge and get to work drinking it. When it's empty, go grab the next one out of the refrigerator, and repeat. Then do it again until you've reached your daily goal.

Personally, I like to hit my water goals with the help of RTIC stainless steel bottles which you can find very reasonably priced at rticcoolers.com. The impressive thing about these jugs is they can hold cold (and hot) temperatures for a long time, and you can get them in sizes ranging from 16-ounces to as large as one-gallon. So, there's never an excuse not to meet your daily water intake.

Strive to log your water intake into whatever calorie-tracking app you use as a way of keeping track of how much you're drinking. Another option is to ask one of your friends to send you a text checking in on your water consumption at various points throughout the day. You can even schedule water breaks in your calendar, set alarms on your phone, or add "drink water" to your daily task list.

Keep in mind that tea (not including herbal teas), coffee, and alcohol are all very dehydrating fluids. They are great to enjoy every once in a while, but they are not meant to replace water when trying to reach your daily fluid goals.

You'll know you're sufficiently hydrated when you're thinking clearly, are full of energy, hit the restroom regularly, sweat easily, and when your urine is a pale yellow.

There are some really excellent benefits to being completely hydrated. Probably one of the best benefits that is quickly noticed is an increase in energy as well as more clear thinking. Water helps to distribute essential nutrients to cells within your body, and it flushes out toxins.

You should be pooping regularly, too, so if you aren't, you need to increase the amount of water you're drinking (and eat more veggies)! Water will quickly clear up constipation issues. I know it seems counterintuitive, but if you're feeling bloated or like you're retaining fluids, drinking more water will eliminate that problem, as well.

I have teenage daughters who love to drink soda. When their skin is breaking out, I remind them that increasing their water consumption and eliminating the soda pop will do wonders to clear up their complexion. It does work, not to mention it gives them a healthy glow.

It is possible, though rare, to drink too much water and create a mineral imbalance in the body, as I mentioned before has happened to me. Sometimes, if this happens, it is because there is an underlying health issue, such as poor adrenal function that causes the body to lack the ability to maintain a state of balance. Likewise, if there is reduced kidney function, there could be water-consumption limits as well.

In case you're curious, an electrolyte is made up of minerals. These minerals are *sodium, potassium, magnesium,* and *chloride.* All help to keep the body's acid levels in check, the muscles contracting, and the nervous system functioning optimally.

Sodium is the electrolyte that is problematic when drinking too much water. Too much liquid dilutes the sodium in our bloodstream and can cause symptoms of bloating or nausea in mild cases. If it's severe, you'll experience fatigue, weakness, feel unsteady, irritable, confused, or even have convulsions. The sodium is responsible for regulating the balance of fluid in each cell.

If adrenal fatigue is something you suffer with or you suspect it to be a problem, try adding a pinch of Himalayan or Celtic Sea Salt to your drinking water. This will offer your body support in maintaining the delicate balance of minerals.

Potassium is another electrolyte that can become depleted. Eating a diet rich in fresh vegetables and enjoying a moderate intake of fruit is an excellent way to take preventative action. Low potassium can result in muscle cramps and heart palpitations, so if you're noticing those symptoms, a banana and a tall glass of water may be just what you need to feel better.

Some fitness lovers like to reach for Gatorade after a workout or when they finish running an event such as a Tough Mudder or Half Marathon. However, I wouldn't encourage that choice of drink at all. It is nothing more than chemicals, sugar, and food coloring.

Instead, I suggest reaching for nature's Gatorade – all-natural coconut water! A small container of it has as much potassium as four bananas! It is high in natural sugar; however, you can dilute it with your regular drinking water to reduce your sugar consumption, which is what I tend to do for myself. It is also an excellent source of energy as a pre-workout drink!

If you're not drinking enough water, you'll know it. Here are the symptoms you'll likely experience if you're dehydrated:

- Depression
- Fatigue
- Water retention
- Dry, sticky mouth
- Sleepiness
- Dry skin
- Headaches
- Dizziness or light-headedness
- Constipation
- Muscle cramps
- Irritability
- Minimal urine output
- Rapid heartbeat and breathing

If you're not enjoying a glass of water yet after reading this section, as your health coach, I encourage you to go pour a tall glass now and get busy drinking it while we move into the subjects of home-cooking and the essential nutrients your body needs to thrive.

Understanding Nutrition in the Kitchen

When I was in my early twenties, I couldn't cook a good meal to save my soul. Even though I had grown up watching and helping my mom in the kitchen, I just never really embraced the joy of cooking. It seemed no matter how hard I tried to cook, I failed at it. Nothing ever turned out right or tasted very good. I was the girl who would neglect to read the recipe all the way through before I started. Three steps in I'd already somehow screwed it up.

I guess it's true that wisdom comes with age because I've finally figured out the kitchen aspect of health and wellness, thank goodness! I had never fully understood the importance of knowing how to plan, prep, and cook tasty and high-quality home-cooked meals until that unexpected thyroiditis hit me. It was then that I discovered how food is like medicine, and when implemented consistently, it would nourish my body back to optimal health.

Did you catch what I just said?

Eating the RIGHT foods was a critical factor
in returning my health to normal.

Using nutrition and implementing lifestyle changes helped me completely heal my thyroid, medication-free, within two years. Not gonna lie. It was tough! In the heat of the struggle, I learned a few valuable lessons.

1. I learned how to eat according to my body's nutritional needs rather than grabbing the first thing I saw or craved. The wrong foods made me feel worse. It was the motivation I needed to make healthier choices.
2. I learned how various foods affected my energy levels, digestion, brain function, quality of sleep, level of endurance, hormones, skin, hair, nails, and even my libido. I began to understand that food was robust fuel for my inner fire.
3. I learned that proper nutrition is powerful – *food is medicine!*

Adequate nutrition is a significant source of fuel for your fire. When your body is well-nourished, you are less likely to be overweight, inactive, sick, or experience various symptoms of imbalance. You'll have abundant energy and a glow about you that is hard to miss. For your body to be in a state of optimal health, proper nutrition is necessary, both in quality and in quantity. It's in your best interest to have a clear understanding for what nutrients your body needs to function correctly. Then take action to implement them into your day to day choices.

Maybe you believe you're already eating healthy. You might, in fact, be! Just keep in mind that symptoms of any kind are a sign of a problem in the body, usually stemming from poor dietary choices. Are you struggling with ailments like lack of energy, forgetfulness, or severe PMS? If so, your diet could use a slight overhaul. Believe me, I didn't think my food was all that bad either until my health (and my training) taught me otherwise. There's so much contradictory information around the subject of nutrition. It *can* be confusing!

When I attended the Institute for Integrative Nutrition®, I had my eyes opened to more than one hundred different dietary theories. Some of them, like the baby food diet, the French women don't get fat diet, and the peanut butter diet actually made me laugh.

Others you've no doubt heard of are Paleo, Ketogenic, Mediterranean, Weight Watchers, Atkins, DASH, and Zone diets. I'm only scraping the surface by mentioning these, as there are countless diets to choose from. It's no wonder people are confused.

Let's talk for a minute about the most popularly consumed diet among most Americans, which is the Standard American Diet (SAD). In this diet 69% of our calories are refined and processed foods, leaving about 25% coming from animal sources and only 6% from fresh vegetables and fruit.

The National Cancer Institute published a report in 2010 showing that three out of four Americans don't eat a single piece of fruit on a given day. Nearly nine out of ten don't reach the daily recommendation of about four servings per day for vegetable consumption. Work with me for any amount of time and you'll quickly learn that eating more vegetables is a non-negotiable. They are so stinking good for you and your body will thank you for them.

For most people, poor diet is an issue of convenience. For others, they just don't know any better. Instead of eating real food, we fill our bodies with artificial chemically-constructed garbage every time we go through the drive-thru window. We order our food from a gas station, reheat processed frozen dinners, and snack on various boxed or bagged foods out of our pantry.

We are practically gorging ourselves with portion sizes large enough to feed a family of four, and we repeat this behavior day in and day out. It's no wonder Americans are dying sooner. We have higher rates of heart disease, cancer, diabetes, autoimmune disease, and obesity than other nations.

According to the World Health Organization, over 80% of chronic disease is preventable through diet and lifestyle choices. That's a pretty impressive number that puts our health right smack in our own hands. I've said it before and it's worth saying again, you hold the power to change your life and your health. You simply have to decide that it matters and why. Then you need to act on making changes.

I realize you may not fully know where to begin, and understandably so! There's a ton of confusion among many about what's okay to eat and what should be avoided. I'm sure you've had your own understanding of how nutrition works, but you may be surprised to learn that some of the old-school ways of looking at nutrition are really not accurate at all.

Go to Amazon and do a search on nutrition, and you'll find hundreds of books published on that topic in 2018 alone! Books and diets intend to solve one problem or another, and in many cases, they do help! The problem is they aren't necessarily sustainable long-term. They also may not be very easy or cost-efficient to follow. And, everybody's body is different, so there is no one diet that works well for everyone. One person's food can be another person's poison. What works for me, may or may not work for you.

So, what makes the advice I'm about to give you any more valid than another expert opinion out there?

Two reasons:

1. I'm not going to teach you a diet. I will give you guidance on how to eat in a way that adequately nourishes your body and your life. Life nourishment is every bit as important, if not more important, than body nourishment. This may require some adjustments in your typical day-to-day choices, especially if you eat and live like most Americans do.
2. I respect the fact that it's your body and your life. You get to be the expert for yourself, which is how it should be. I'll give you the knowledge and the tools for fueling your fire. It's up to you to tune into your body and your life, try new things, and learn what works best for you. Then once you know what helps you to thrive, keep doing it. It's your perfect lifestyle!

Home cooking is one of the easiest ways to start immediately improving your health. I always like to say *"nutrition matters"* because it does. When you feed your body food that it recognizes, it functions much more efficiently. Preservatives, chemicals, and excessive amounts of processed sugar will only slow your body down.

Sure, a candy bar now and then won't kill you. The cheeseburger you grabbed for lunch at Burger King won't make you sick right this moment. Those choices add up over time, though, and that's why we seem to start falling apart around the third or fourth decade of life.

The cumulative effect processed foods and refined sugars have on our body eventually causes the liver and other organs to get overloaded. The big problem with this is our liver is responsible for so many vital functions that help to keep us thriving. One role, in particular, is removing excess estrogen from the body. If the liver isn't working optimally, this can create hormone problems. Once there is a hormone imbalance, a downward spiral effect can occur with your health.

Your liver is also responsible for processing all of the sugar you're consuming. The quickest way to turn your body into a fat-storage machine is to overeat sugar. If your belly, hips, butt, or thighs have been growing, it would be wise to pay attention to how much sugar you're consuming, even if you think you aren't eating much of it at all. More on that later.

Keep in mind, however, if you're already in the mess of a health problem, proper nutrition is not a quick fix. It's not like taking a pill, and *POOF*, your symptoms are all gone. You didn't get sick overnight. Getting better will take time and a change in lifestyle. The results don't happen overnight. When you eat the right food for your body, you will notice a gradual difference in how you feel.

This same concept holds with weight loss as well. You didn't gain weight overnight. You will not lose it overnight, and it will require a reasonable, solid effort of consistently making real food choices along with proper exercise.

I hate to be the bearer of bad news, but there is no such thing as healthy restaurant food. It doesn't matter if it's fast food or a fancy sit-down restaurant. Both are businesses, and for a company to be profitable, expenses must be controlled. This typically means skimping on quality to get a higher quantity of ingredients at a much lower price.

Aim to source 90% of your meals from home-cooking. While you can still find some healthy options when dining out, it is much more challenging to do. When you choose to prepare your meals at home, you put the power of your health into your own hands. You get to control the quality of the ingredients you use, and the portion sizes you serve. You also get to feel proud of what you've created and customize the flavors to your preference. Home cooking is often more budget friendly as well, even if you're purchasing higher quality ingredients.

SECRET #10

Get Started with Home Cooking

Home cooking is not always the most convenient option. I'll give you that! Recently one of my clients requested information on how to avoid starting her meals on fire and accidentally burning down her kitchen. She was joking, I hope. But the point is, cooking isn't everyone's gift, and if you have small children or pets underfoot it can be exasperating. With a little bit of planning, it really isn't all that difficult, though. At the end of this book you'll find a handful of healthy recipes you can try out as you venture into more frequent home-cooked meals.

To get started, begin by creating a simple meal plan for one week. Look at your calendar and see what you have going on in the evening hours around dinner time. If you have something going on that keeps you out of the house until late, consider doing an easy crockpot meal that day. It will be cooking while you're out of the house and is simple to dish up as soon as you walk in the door.

There are a lot of quick, simple, and healthy meal ideas you can consider, and there is nothing wrong with repetition if it gets you away from dining out or eating processed junk. You can always add variety later, once you've established a new routine. It's perfectly okay to keep it simple in the beginning.

Here is how I often keep things simple in my own home cooking.

- Breakfast is almost always two eggs over-medium with a side of vegetables, or an apple with Greek yogurt and raw cacao nibs or chia seeds sprinkled over the top.
- Lunch is usually a nice big veggie salad. Soaking and cooking beans at the beginning of the week make an excellent protein addition to salad, and so does a hard-boiled egg or grilled chicken breast prepared during your weekly food prep session.
- For dinner, I always start with a protein source and add lots of fresh vegetables on the side. Sometimes I like to add quinoa or brown rice as well. Since those take longer to prepare, I plan ahead and make them when I know I'll be home while they simmer on the stove. Then I just quickly reheat them when I'm ready for them. (By the way, I discovered I really love making brown rice porridge for breakfast with leftover rice. It is so tasty!)
- Fruit makes a perfect dessert for a sweet tooth. Try grilling or baking it! Yum!

Healthy and straightforward go-to meals you can add to your meal plan right away are:

- **Grilled chicken breasts.** I purchase thin breasts, so they cook quicker on my countertop smokeless grill.
- **Oven-baked chicken thighs.** These cook up nicely in only about 20 minutes or so and are delicious – and cheap!
- **Grass-fed burgers** are ready to eat in 10-15 minutes. I cut fresh potatoes into fries, shake them in a bag with a healthy oil, and roast them on a cookie sheet at 4250F until they're brown. They are usually ready by the time the burgers are cooked. I even like to make my own burger buns when time allows. Homemade bread products are much healthier than store-bought, even if you are using white flour. The reason is your homemade bread won't have the preservatives or chemicals store-bought bread has. You can also buy higher-quality organic, unbleached flour.

- **Chuck roast in the crockpot**. You need at least 3 hours of slow cooking time. I toss in some onion, carrots, red cooking wine, organic beef bone broth, and a few sprigs of rosemary. Delicious!
- **Homemade tacos**. Quick and so simple. I even mix my own taco seasoning to avoid unnecessary chemicals from packaged taco seasoning. I prefer not to eat the store-bought taco shells, so I usually make my meal a taco salad instead. Place taco meat, cheese, salsa, avocado, and sour cream over a bed of raw spinach. Easy peasy!

Cooking at home doesn't have to be complicated, and it is so much healthier than dining out. I use my crockpot and my countertop grill for almost everything! It's about progress, not perfection. The most crucial step is just to decide you want to be healthier and that you want it for your family, too! Then put your decision into action. Every little bit helps!

Also, be mindful of your eating habits by making each meal pleasurable, satiating, and nourishing. This helps to create a healthy mindset shift that will lead you to success in your overall lifestyle choices.

To Make Your Meals More Pleasurable:

Take the time to prepare your meal with love and a positive attitude. Smell the aroma. Invite an awesome friend to join you. Experiment with new foods, different seasonings, change your cooking method or try an original recipe to keep things exciting. Arrange it on the plate in a fun, fancy way. Have fun with this! Take a picture and share it on your favorite social media platform. Be proud of your creation and thoroughly enjoy every bite.

To Make Your Meals More Satiating:

Don't be afraid of a little bit of fat. Healthy fats like olive oil, avocado oil, grass-fed butter, or coconut oil can make a meal taste so delicious and satisfying. Don't deprive your body of high quality, whole foods for the sake of reducing calories. This will only lead to hunger and binging later. When you eat, take your time. Chew slowly. Try to get the food to near liquid in your mouth before you swallow. This is very beneficial for healthy digestion.

To Make Your Meals More Nourishing:

Eat real food. Be aware of how your body responds to the food you eat and honor your body by avoiding what doesn't agree with it. If you eat something and then immediately have a reaction to it like it flushes right through you, or you have gas and bloating, it's not a food that agrees with your body, so avoid it in the future or try a different method of preparation. For example: soaking your beans before you cook them. The human body is incredibly intelligent, and it sends signals when something is causing it to work much harder.

Confession Time

Cookies are my weakness! If they're in the house, I'll eat them. If they're on a table at a party, I'll eat them. If they're anywhere in my line of sight and are readily available to eat, I'll eat them. I can do everything else right when it comes to food choices but offer me a cookie and all hell breaks loose because I can't stop with just one. Throw in a tall glass of creamy, whole chocolate milk to dunk those cookies in, and you definitely hold the secret for taking me down!

I just wanted you to know that even though nutrition is 80% of my business, I face temptations too and I'm not always perfect in my choices. I avoid feelings of deprivation by eating really well and by following the 90/10 rule, as mentioned earlier. I do, indeed, allow myself the opportunity to splurge every so often.

SECRET #11

Eat Real, Nutrient-Dense Foods

What if I told you to eat whatever your heart desires, as long as each meal contains a high-quality source of protein, some healthy fat, and a side of vegetables? What if I also told you never to skip a meal and to drink plenty of water throughout the day?

Does that seem too restrictive or too challenging to achieve? It shouldn't. I'm not even giving you specific grams of each to stick to. At least, not yet. Eating healthy should not come with a side of anxiety, overwhelm, or deprivation.

Depending on your current choices and lifestyle, it could still be a hard change for you. For most, if there's a plan in place and the food prep has been done before the week begins, this method of eating is extremely doable. It's also healthy and won't ever leave you feeling deprived or hungry! The beauty of it is, *you* get to choose what you eat. I'm not making that decision for you. Doesn't it feel nice to know you have the power here? You get to make decisions that are best for your unique body!

But here's the key to having that choice – you need to be willing to follow my guidance and feed your body the *right* way, even if you don't like a particular food group, like vegetables, for example.

For your body to thrive and survive, you must provide it with adequate levels of protein, complex carbohydrates (vegetables and whole grains), and healthy fats from clean sources. When you choose high-quality ingredients, along with focusing on improving your gut health, which I'll discuss more later, you'll take in all the vitamins and minerals your body needs.

If you've been eating a ton of processed foods and refined sugar, you may find that a change in your food choices will instill a natural cleansing process. As your body detoxifies, minor symptoms may occur. These symptoms will dissipate as you continue to put clean, real food into your body. Be sure to drink 1/2 your body weight in ounces of water per day and get plenty of rest to help your body adequately detox.

Once the detox symptoms lessen, it won't take long for you to know you're doing something right because you'll start to feel freaking amazing! Trust the process and keep going.

Power Up with Protein

If you love eating a juicy steak or find that you have cravings for salmon, cheese, or nuts, I have great news for you. You get to enjoy these foods whenever you like! Consuming enough high-quality protein is something I encourage all of my clients to do daily, and in fact, with each meal.

Every cell in your body contains protein, so meeting your protein requirement is essential to your health. Proteins are made up of amino acids. Twenty are found in the human body, but our body only produces 11 on its own. The other 9 are essential because we don't make them, so we need to get them from food sources.

Your body uses protein to build and repair tissues. You also use protein for proper immune function, to make enzymes, and to create hormones. Protein is an essential building block of bones, muscles, cartilage, skin, and blood. Thankfully, getting adequate sources of protein through the food we eat isn't usually too hard to do.

However, if you don't have enough protein in your body, you can experience any or all of these wide range of symptoms:

- Edema (swollen, puffy skin)
- Fatty liver (fat accumulation in liver cells)
- Skin, hair, and nail problems
- Loss of muscle mass
- Greater risk of bone fractures
- Increased severity of infections
- Greater appetite and calorie intake

Not everyone has the same protein requirements, so I can't tell you exactly how much protein you should be consuming on any given day. It depends on your weight, muscle mass, activity levels, and age. You can look at the RDA (recommended daily allowance) as a general rule of thumb to follow.

The RDA suggests 0.4 grams of protein for each pound of body weight. So, for example, a 165-pound adult would need at least 66 grams of protein per day. Athletes, or those who exercise a lot, should be consuming closer to 0.5 to 0.6 grams for each pound of body weight. But I've seen recommendations even as high as 0.9 grams of protein per pound of body weight. Most of us need about 10-35% of our total caloric intake from protein. If you are sick, pregnant, aging, or are doing intense physical activity, your protein needs will be more significant.

It's really up to you how much protein you consume. Always listen to your body and pay attention to things like how healthy your nails are, how much energy you have, how satiated you feel after meals, how strong your muscles recover from workouts, and even if you're losing a lot of hair or it's thinning. While you can get too much protein for your kidneys to process, it's not typically an issue unless you are already having problems with your kidney function.

Aiming for a high amount of protein with each meal is always a great start, and I would even consider adding in a protein shake after a workout, and snacks that are high-quality sources of protein as well.

Some great sources of protein you can include in your diet regularly are:

Protein Sources					
Soybeans	Eggs	Sunflower Seeds	Oats	Cheddar Cheese	Beef
Kidney Beans	Almonds	Chia Seeds	Cottage Cheese	Greek Yogurt	Tuna
Chickpeas	Pistachios	Turkey Breast	Parmesan Cheese	Kefir	Quinoa
Pumpkin Seeds	Cashews & Peanuts	Salmon	Swiss Cheese	Milk	High-Quality Whey Protein
Flax Seeds	Chicken Breast	Shrimp	Mozzarella Cheese	Broccoli & Brussel Sprouts	Lentils

If you're a vegetarian or vegan and don't eat meat, you'll still be fine. Just choose a wide variety of the options noted above.

Power Up with Healthy Fats

Too many folks these days are afraid of eating fats, and they shouldn't be. Fats are necessary fuel in our diets for achieving and maintaining energy and also for optimal health. The low-fat and non-fat trend these past few decades are actually a big fat nutrition lie that has been fed to the public.

It's time for fats to stop having a bad rap. None of the studies that have been done have actually linked high-fat diets to heart disease. It's the quality and type of fat eaten that plays a significant role in our health.

By not eating enough fat, you're actually doing yourself a disservice, as some fats help balance hormones and reduce the risk of heart attack.

From a weight-loss perspective, fat is satiating, and so you won't be hungry as quickly in between meals, nor will you feel deprived. Fats also help absorb fat-soluble vitamins. Supporting brain development, providing cushioning and insulation to internal organs, and playing a significant role in hormone creation are other ways fat helps us. At 9 calories per gram, fats are the highest energy source per gram of the three macronutrients.

Visit other parts of the world, and you'll see that fat is always welcome at the table. There was a study done in the New England Journal of Medicine that found a high fat and low carb diet aids weight loss and reduces cholesterol.

Guess what? Your body actually needs fat, particularly the healthy fats, to function correctly. Good fats lower cholesterol levels, boost brain function, and help to keep you satiated so you don't overeat. Fat keeps your hair and skin healthy, supplies energy, and helps regulate your body temperature.

So, what is considered healthy fat versus unhealthy fat?

Monounsaturated fatty acids are heart-healthy and support LDL (bad) and HDL (good) cholesterol levels. These fats tend to be liquid at room temperature. Monounsaturated fats are your Omega 9s and are the most abundant fats in most cells in the body. They can be produced by the body and therefore are not "essential fatty acids". They're common in nut and seed oils, and plant oils such as avocado oil and olive oil.

Polyunsaturated fatty acids are essential to consume because your body is unable to produce them on its own. They are Omega-3 and Omega-6 fatty acids. Omega-3 fatty acids are necessary for reducing inflammation in your body, supporting your heart health, reducing symptoms of depression, and reducing cancer risk.

There are many types of omega-3 fats, which differ based on their chemical shape and size. Here are the three most common:

- Eicosapentaenoic acid (EPA): Their main function is to produce chemicals called eicosanoids, which help reduce inflammation. EPA also helps reduce symptoms of depression.
- Docosahexaenoic acid (DHA): DHA makes up about 8% of brain weight and is extremely important for normal brain development and function.
- Alpha-linolenic acid (ALA): This fatty acid is mainly used by the body for energy.

Omega-3 fats are a crucial part of human cell membranes and can be found in oily fatty fish such as salmon, tuna, mackerel, herring, anchovies, and sardines, flax seeds and chia seeds.

It's essential for you to have both Omega-3's and Omega-6's, but it's easier to get Omega 6 fats, found in eggs, corn, sunflower oil, soybeans (used in many processed foods), meat, poultry, and nuts and seeds. The ratio definitely needs to favor the Omega-3's as too much Omega-6 actually promotes inflammation.

Saturated fatty acids tend to be considered unhealthy fats because they are associated with obesity and cardiovascular disease.

Many people – including health and medical professionals – think coconut oil falls into the bad fat category because it's a saturated fat, but that simply isn't the case. Coconut oil is a plant-based source of saturated fat that, unlike animal-based sources, is high in lauric acid and has beneficial antibacterial, anti-fungal, and even cholesterol-lowering properties.

Trans fatty acids are the result of hydrogenation and have a high association with the hardening of the arteries and heart disease. Watch nutrition labels for the words partially hydrogenated, which means trans fats are present. These are very inflammatory fats and should be avoided at all costs. They can be found in many peanut butters, bakery products, some microwaveable popcorn, fast fried foods, some margarines, non-dairy coffee creamers, and snack foods such as potato and corn chips, meat pies and sausage rolls, and some crackers. This is not a definitive list.

The U.S. Food and Drug Administration (FDA) banned trans fats in 2015, giving manufacturers three years to eliminate them, with a deadline of June 18, 2018. You should no longer see them on grocery store shelves, but be alert anyway.

It is wise to limit your consumption of saturated fats from animal sources to 10% or less of your total calories consumed. Targeting 20-35% or more of your daily energy needs from healthy fats will go a long way in promoting an optimally healthy, thriving body and weight loss, too. That doesn't mean you can never eat butter again, for example, but if you love butter, eat pastured butter (and all animal products for that matter, if you can). It may be difficult to find where you live, but Kerrigold brand Irish butter is one source of pastured butter. And it says so right on the label.

Healthy Fat Sources	
Avocados	Fatty Wild Caught Fish
Grass-Fed Butter	Nuts
Ghee	Organic, Pastured Eggs
Organic Coconut Oil	Grass-fed Beef
Extra-Virgin Olive Oil	Seeds

Power Up with Complex Carbohydrates

People often think carbs are fattening foods. But complex carbohydrates, like whole grains, are not. It's the type and quantity of the carbs you eat – not the carbohydrates themselves – that cause weight gain. The right kind of carbohydrates in your diet will give you usable fuel, or energy, to promote healthy digestion and a healthy weight.

High-quality carbohydrates like whole grains and vegetables are perfect choices for a busy, active lifestyle. The refined carbs are the ones you want to watch out for, as these increase risk for chronic inflammation, obesity, and type 2 diabetes.

It's helpful to understand that there are two types of carbs: Simple and Complex.

Simple carbs break down quickly, providing a fast burst of energy. Complex carbs require more time to break down, slowing digestion and absorption, which prevents extreme changes in blood sugar levels.

Simple carbs are things like fruit, honey, glucose, sugar, malt sugar (maltose), and dairy (lactose). *Fruit is a natural source of sugar, but also a good source of fiber, vitamins, minerals, and antioxidants that are all great for your health. It is still sugar, though. Don't avoid fruit, but instead be cautious not to over-consume it.

Eat Plenty of These Carbohydrates

High Quality Complex Carbohydrates			
Brown Rice & Wild Rice	Beans	Apples	Cucumbers
Whole Oats	Legumes	Nuts & Seeds	Peppers
Whole Wheat	Root Vegetables	Fresh Herbs	Squash
Barley, Bulgur, Buckwheat	Leafy Green Vegetables	Quinoa	Tomatoes

All of these foods are loaded with fiber, so they help support cardiovascular health and a healthy weight. Avoid refined grains that no longer contain fiber such as white flour.

A note about potatoes: everyone thinks potatoes are best to be avoided, but they aren't. The only potatoes you should avoid are those that come served in a McDonald's (or other fast food restaurant) container. Home-cooked potatoes using healthy oils or grass-fed butter are incredibly nutritious! They are loaded with potassium, fiber, and vitamin C. Be sure to eat the skin, too!

The RDA for carbohydrates is 45-65% of your total calories. To make your diet as nutrient dense as possible, the majority of your carbs should come from vegetables and whole food sources, not refined grains or added sugars.

Carbohydrates to Avoid

Refined Carbohydrates and Sugars		
White Bread, including Bagels	Pretzels	Muffins & Cookies
White Rice	Candy	Juice
White Pasta	Soda & Beer	Flavored Yogurt
Chips	Ice Cream & Cakes	Energy Bars
Crackers	Breakfast Cereals	Specialty Coffee Drinks

These are all considered to be refined carbs, or they are stripped of the outside grain, which makes glucose levels spike quickly. When choosing which carbs to eat, always look at how nutrient-dense it is first. Is it high in fiber? Is it high in protein? If so, then it's probably a great choice!

The Power of Vegetables

When was the last time you enjoyed some leafy greens?

As an Integrative Nutrition Health Coach, I get a 'bird's eye view' into a typical daily diet for most of my clients or potential clients. Many of them reach out to me to either lose weight or balance their hormones. They tell me they pretty much already eat "healthy." What they are looking for is some guidance and accountability to resolve their specific health struggles, which I'm happy to help with.

During a health consultation, one of the first things I discover is the lack of leafy green vegetables (and in some cases the absence of *any* plants) in the average person's diet. By the way, just so you know, corn is not a vegetable. It is a grain. Green beans and peas are legumes.

It's no secret that vegetables – leafy greens, in particular – are super healthy for us! Unfortunately, most people are missing out on the nutritional power leafy greens provide.

Getting into the habit of consuming more leafy greens in your diet is essential for a healthy body and immune system. Once you start to nourish our body with greens, you'll begin the process of crowding out foods that make you sick. It's really one of the best choices you can make for your long term health and wellness.

There are numerous benefits to eating more leafy green vegetables!

Greens are really good at strengthening our blood and respiratory system. The darker the shade, the more potent the anti-inflammatory agents are that are present in them. Vitamin C and beta-carotene are a few examples of anti-inflammatories present in dark leafy vegetables. Leafy greens, when consumed with foods rich in vitamin C, are a great source of iron. The vitamin C helps improve absorption.

Leafy greens are also highly alkaline, which is beneficial for those living in polluted urban areas. For those looking to reduce their risk of cancer, and those who struggle with symptoms of an acidic system, eating more veggies will help restore the pH balance in your blood and cells! Green vegetables also help replenish our alkaline mineral stores.

Kale, the king of greens, is a good source of omega fatty acids. Nutritionally speaking, leafy greens are high in calcium, magnesium, iron, potassium, and vitamins A, C, & K. They are also loaded with fiber and folic acid, as well as chlorophyll.

Fun Fact:

The color green is associated with Spring, which is a time of renewal, refreshment, and energy. To add to this fascinating theory, in Traditional Chinese Medicine, the color green is related to the liver, emotional stability, and creativity. Pretty cool, eh?

There are other proven and possible benefits of consuming leafy greens such as blood purification, cancer prevention, improved circulation, strengthened immune system, promotion of healthy intestinal flora or gut bacteria, improved liver, gallbladder, kidney function, and cleared congestion, especially in the lungs, by reducing mucus.

When grocery shopping, try to buy organic greens. If that's not possible, then consume them non-organic. It will be okay. Just get vegetables into your body. You won't regret doing so.

There's a wide variety of greens to choose from, keeping your own unique body and needs in mind. If you've been told to avoid cruciferous veggies for health reasons, listen to your doctor. If you know a particular green doesn't agree with you, avoid it.

Enjoy a wide variety of these leafy greens in your meals

Examples of Healthy Greens			
Broccoli	Bok Choy	Napa Cabbage	Kale
Collards	Watercress	Mustard Greens	Dandelion Greens
Green Cabbage (cooked, raw, or as sauerkraut)	Arugula	Chicory	Lettuce
Endive	Spinach	Swiss Chard	Beet Greens

*Note: Enjoy spinach, Swiss chard, and beet greens in moderation, as they are high in oxalic acid which can interfere with the absorption of calcium.

These all have incredible health benefits of their own, so don't avoid them altogether. Rotating between a variety of leafy green vegetables shouldn't cause any nutritional deficiencies related to calcium.

**One other side note: if you have a thyroid problem, it's best to avoid eating cruciferous vegetables raw. A little here and there shouldn't be cause for alarm but enjoying them cooked will be much better for your particular health concerns.

The more nutrient dense your food is, the better nourished your body will be and the more satiated you'll feel after meals.

The most nutrient-dense foods to consume

If you want to function optimally and feel amazing, these are the best foods to incorporate into your weekly meal planning. Always remember the more variety in your diet, the more your body will benefit from a vast array of vitamins, antioxidants, and minerals. Be sure to consume enough healthy fats, especially if you're super active. Too much fiber and not enough calories can actually damage your health rather than be a benefit. Everything in variety and moderation, right?

Most Nutrient-Dense Foods				
Seaweed	Tomatoes	Liver	Kale, Collards and Dandelion Greens	Broccoli
Exotic berries: Acai, Goji, Camu Camu	Wild Mushrooms	Spinach, Watercress, Arugula	Cauliflower	Cabbage
Red Peppers	Seeds: Pumpkin, Sunflower, Chia, Flax	Garlic & Parsley	Avocados	Berries: Blueberries, Raspberries, Blackberries
Asparagus	Raw Cheese & Kefir	Carrots	Beets	Wild-Caught Salmon
Bone Broth	Sweet Potatoes	Grass-fed beef & Venison	Green Beans	Egg Yolks
Brown Rice & Wild Rice	Black Beans	Pumpkin	Lentils	Artichokes

SECRET #12

Supplement Where Needed

I know it may seem tempting just to take a vitamin or some fancy supplements in the place of healthy food. However, I must plead with you to avoid that way of thinking. Your nutrition really should come, first and foremost, from the foods you eat.

If malabsorption is a problem for you, which is sometimes the case with thyroid conditions or gut dysbiosis, then it's a good idea to supplement beyond your meals. This is especially vital if you've traditionally eaten the SAD way for years with no vitamins to support your body.

It's not within my scope of practice to prescribe any particular supplements for you to take. I am, however, knowledgeable in what the body needs for proper nourishment, so take this information for what it is – suggestions for you to consider or explore with your own healthcare team.

You are your body's own best expert. If you do add in any new supplements, I would add them in one at a time and watch for symptoms that indicate a potential problem or allergic response. My role is simply to empower you to be informed and to act in the best interest of your own health through the proper channels.

Vitamins That Will Fuel Your Hottest Fire

VITAMIN A: A fat-soluble vitamin, essential for skin and bones. The body uses it as an antioxidant, and it also helps to produce hormones that are involved in gene regulation.

Good food sources are animal liver, grass-fed butter and dairy products, grass-fed meat and poultry, sweet potato, cantaloupe, carrots and other orange foods, and dark leafy greens.

VITAMIN B12: A water-soluble vitamin, necessary for proper neurological function and red blood cell formation. You can find this in animal products in its natural form. Deficiency can be a problem for those on acid-blocker meds, those with inflammation of the small intestine, and those who have autoimmune conditions.

Good food sources are grass-fed beef and beef liver, wild-caught fish, lamb, and eggs.

VITAMIN D: Vitamin D is actually a fat-soluble hormone produced by the kidneys. Vitamin D synthesis is generated when the skin is exposed to sunlight. Having enough of this vitamin allows for calcium absorption in the gut and helps to maintain adequate levels of calcium in the body which is good for healthy bones. It's also a big player in regulating hormones. Unfortunately, when there is inflammation in the body, vitamin D deficiency is usually a factor. Increasing vitamin D through sunlight and diet are the first steps to getting healthier. Because this is a fat-soluble vitamin, you do need to exercise caution when supplementing because you can get too much of it. Always check with your doctor to see if you need it before adding a supplement.

Good food sources are fatty wild-caught fish, such as salmon, tuna, and mackerel, cod liver or cod liver oil, eggs and dairy products.

VITAMIN K2: This vitamin works closely with vitamin D. You need adequate levels of vitamin K2 for Vitamin D to function properly. K2 is essential for bone strength and blood vessels. It is also crucial for a healthy pregnancy.

Good food sources are fermented foods like kimchi, sauerkraut, natto, yogurt, and raw grass-fed dairy.

IRON: This is a trace element most bioavailable through animal food sources. It is also present in plant sources, but those are much more difficult to break down into a usable form. Eating something high in vitamin C with a plant source of iron will help with absorption. If you're noticing fatigue, weakness, pale skin, lightheadedness, hair loss, dizziness, or headaches, it might be a good idea to have your doctor check your iron levels. Deficiency is widespread in women due to menstruation.

Good food sources are animal liver, lean meats (venison, in particular), seafood, beans, nuts, and veggies.

IODINE: This is another trace element, and it's necessary for proper thyroid function. Most people get their iodine from eating iodized salt. However, there has been gaining popularity of sea salt and Himalayan salt instead, which are not iodized. Therefore, iodine deficiencies are becoming more common. If you are experiencing a thyroid imbalance, a natural healthcare practitioner may suggest iodine supplementation. This is very controversial, and caution should be used when taking any kind of supplements. I personally have used iodine supplements in my own health journey with absolutely no problems and actually improved my health without the need for medication. Everyone's body and circumstances are different, though. Do your research and become your own health advocate.

Good food sources are seaweed, seafood, dairy, and eggs.

MAGNESIUM: This is a vital mineral often referred to as nature's relaxation mineral. It does a lot for our health, but one thing in particular is maintaining blood sugar balance. Those with type 2 diabetes and PCOS might benefit from having their magnesium levels checked for deficiency. Magnesium is excellent for hormone balance, inducing sleep, and reducing symptoms of anxiety.

Good food sources to reach for are leafy greens, avocados, seaweed, beans, nuts, pumpkin seeds, sunflower seeds, and sesame seeds.

OMEGA-3 FATTY ACIDS: This is an essential fatty acid because the body cannot make it on its own, so getting it through food or supplements is a good idea. The best sources are found in oily fatty fish because it's harder for the body to use it in a plant-based form. Omega-3 reduces inflammation in the body and helps to prevent heart disease, diabetes, and autoimmune conditions.

Good food sources are wild-caught fish, such as salmon, mackerel, sardines, and herring. Walnuts, chia seeds, and flax-seeds.

FOLATE (B9): This vitamin is necessary for building red blood cells and maintaining DNA function. Folate is the natural form of B9 (not folic acid) and is the type most preferred by the body. If you suffer from chronic low energy, anemia, or mouth sores, it's worth exploring whether or not you have a deficiency.

Good food sources are spinach, cruciferous veggies like Brussel sprouts and asparagus, beans, peas, avocado, and beef liver.

VITAMIN C: This is a water-soluble vitamin that acts as an antioxidant and helps with maintaining the health of the body's connective tissues. It is also suitable for your heart and hormones specifically related to adrenal health. It regulates the synthesis of the structural protein collagen. One other important factor is that vitamin C aids in the absorption of other nutrients in the body.

Good food sources are red pepper, kiwi, guava, green bell pepper, oranges, strawberries, papaya, broccoli, kale, parsley, pineapple, Brussels sprouts, cauliflower, mango, lemon, grapefruit, honeydew, peas, and tomatoes.

ZINC: This is an essential trace element and is present in every cell, organ, bone, tissue, and fluid in the body. Even plants and animals need it to survive. Zinc not only aids in a healthy gut lining, but it also helps with hormone balance, a healthy immune system, a rocking sex drive, and more.

Good food sources are pumpkin seeds, grass-fed beef, lamb, cashews, chickpeas, mushrooms, chicken, yogurt, cocoa powder, and spinach.

Watch for Nutrient Deficiencies

Micronutrient deficiencies can occur when our diets are off-balance, and you may not think to look for a deficiency when you're noticing new symptoms. Nutrient deficiencies can actually be detrimental to your body and its ability to function at an optimal state. If you are deficient in nutrients, symptoms will occur causing you to feel off, or just not your best self physically or emotionally, or both.

It is always a good idea to have a CBC (complete blood count) test on yourself once a year to stay on top of what's normal for you. Women should have a full thyroid panel and sex hormone panel if they have any unusual symptoms, but especially once they turn forty, and then regularly after that.

For vitamin deficiency concerns, let your doctor know you'd like a specific vitamin tested so they can order the right tests. By the way, always get a copy of your blood work for your own eyes to see. This is just common sense in being your own health advocate. You know your body better than anyone else does or ever will. If something feels off, it probably is, regardless of what your medical team may be telling you. Having your lab results in your own hands allows you the opportunity to pursue anything in question from a natural approach before it becomes detrimental to your health.

When considering supplementation of a nutrient, keep this in mind: it is always best to get your nutrients from food first. However, in some cases, such as those who have autoimmune struggles or leaky gut, the body may have trouble absorbing nutrients, and therefore supplementation could be helpful.

In situations where absorption is a problem, it's best to treat the root cause first. I suggest working with a knowledgeable professional who understands gut health, such as a functional medicine doctor, or another trained practitioner or nutrition health coach with that specialty. This is something that, based on my training, I do have the ability to help my clients navigate through.

Quantity and Quality Matters

When it comes to vitamins, you can get too much of a good thing. But typically, this is only a problem with fat-soluble vitamins. Those are vitamins A, D, E, K, and iron. Always have your blood levels tested before you supplement beyond the standard multivitamin.

Supplements are a massive industry with an estimated twenty-seven billion dollars in sales every year in the United States alone. Sadly, a lot of companies are just in it for the profits while offering very little quality.

Supplements can contain many ingredients. Some ingredients may not be necessary for your health, or they could be harmful. It's wise to do some research to make sure they won't interact with anything else you're currently taking. Additionally, you want to be sure you won't have an unintended allergic reaction. Hormonal creams and gels, such as testosterone or progesterone and even magnesium oil, are also considered to be supplements.

The FDA doesn't currently regulate supplements at all. It is up to the manufacturer to ensure the product being distributed is safe. They are also responsible for making sure there are no false claims and that it isn't misleading. The product must comply with Federal Food, Drug, and Cosmetic Act and FDA regulations in all other aspects. The FDA also doesn't test or approve supplements unless they feel there is a reason for a particular brand or item.

Qualities to look for in a good supplement are:

- Tested ingredients – the product should have been tested using a randomized trial.
- Bioavailable formula, meaning having a whole food option that is free from preservatives, fillers, dyes, gluten, yeast, and other common allergens.

- A recommended dosage for the benefit that is desired.
- Standardized extracts for herbs and glandulars.
- Also, look for whether or not the product actually contains what it claims to and that the ingredients aren't diluted with other things.
- It's good to have a vegan or vegetarian capsule for people who adhere to those practices.
- It should be a reputable company such as Designs for Health, Standard Process, Pure Encapsulations, Thorne Research, Vital Nutrients, and Gaia Herbs. Other excellent companies I've had great luck with are Metagenics and Nutritional Frontiers.

Supplements that meet these standards are not cheap, but in many cases, you get what you pay for. Medlineplus.gov is an excellent resource for researching any vitamins or supplements you are considering for yourself. This is a government agency, though, so they tend to be very conservative with their recommendations.

There is always a possibility of interactions between supplements and other medications. Consult with your physician before adding in a new supplement or at the very least do your own research to make sure the two will play well together.

I'm often asked the question, "Do vitamins and supplements really work?" My answer is yes, if you get something of high quality and you are deficient in that particular nutrient. You should notice a difference fairly quickly as you start to replenish your need for it. If you don't see a difference, either you're having a hard time absorbing it due to leaky gut, or you're not taking a high-quality brand.

SECRET #13

Crowd out Sugar

Not long ago I sat across the table from a new client as we went over the terms of her program agreement. When we got to the section labeled "Personal Responsibility and Release of Health Care Related Claims" I let her know that she assumes the risks inherent in making lifestyle changes, trying new foods, etc.… then, jokingly, I said, "If, because you've decided to remove all sources of sugar from your home, and your children or your husband retaliate by trying to suffocate you while you're sleeping, that's not on me." We both got a good chuckle out of it, but in all seriousness, sugar is very addictive, and it is something I do suggest slowly crowding out of your diet. Hopefully, your family members will be supportive and not feel the need to go to such extreme measures.

In Nutrition School, I had the privilege of being trained by some of the world's leading experts in health and wellness. Dr. Mark Hyman was one such expert. I recall watching a fascinating lecture from him about the biology of food addiction. One thing that stood out to me most was the topic of sugar. It's so bad for you that it's almost an equivalent to putting poison in your body every time you consume it.

If you could cut or drastically reduce only one thing from your diet today that would make a hugely positive impact on your health, my suggestion would be to kick sugar to the curb.

Sugar is one of the biggest contributors to heart disease, diabetes, cancer, and obesity. A lot of health experts agree that sugar actually feeds cancer. The calorie composition of sugar is super high, we overindulge, and it often ends up being stored as fat if that energy is not used, which leads to obesity. Obesity leads to insulin resistance which increases blood sugar levels and often results in diabetes.

In 2014 there was a large meta-analysis done where they looked at sugar consumption. People who regularly consumed large amounts of sugar, tripled their risk of having a heart attack! That's alarming! What's worse – we are eating poisonous doses of sugar and white flour each year.

In his lecture, Dr. Hyman shared this disturbing fact:

Every person in America consumes an average of 146 pounds of flour and 152 pounds of sugar per year, which is up from only 40 pounds in 1980. That equates to almost one pound per day, per person.

Just let that sink in. If I calculated this correctly, one pound of sugar is somewhere in the ballpark of about 32 tablespoons! Would you dump a little over 10 tablespoons of sugar on your dinner plate at each meal?

That's a pretty powerful visual, isn't it? So how is it possible that we eat so much sugar? I mean, it doesn't look like we do, right? We try to make healthy choices. We aren't loading our dinner plate with pie and cookies only to wash those down with a 32-ounce Dr. Pepper, right?

Sugar is everywhere in some form or another. Food manufacturers are changing the name of it in their ingredient lists to hide the fact that sugar is there because so many people are finally starting to understand how unhealthy it is. Plus, it's *so* highly addictive!

Sugar negatively affects the brain in much the same way as heroin and cocaine. Eating sugar (and doing drugs) creates a surge of the feel-good chemical's dopamine and serotonin. When that surge diminishes, we want to feel it again, and again, and this is how it can quickly become an addiction. One that never fully satisfies. Bad for us. Suitable for food companies looking to create a profit.

Avoid These Sugars*

Sugar/Sucrose	High Fructose Corn Syrup (HFCS)
Agave Nectar	Beet Sugar
Blackstrap Molasses	Brown Sugar
Cane Sugar	Cane Juice Crystals
Confectioner's Sugar	Date Sugar
Evaporated Cane Juice	Florida Crystals
Corn Syrup	Dextrose
Golden Syrup	Maltodextrin
Ethyl Maltol	Brown Rice Syrup
Crystalline Fructose	Fructose
D-ribose	

I'm sorry if this news isn't what you want to hear, but sugar really does need to be crowded out from your diet. Don't think that you aren't eating very much of it. You'd be surprised by how much you're unknowingly consuming every day.

More sobering information:
- Out of 600,000 food products, 80% are made with added sugar.
- 8-15% of our calories often come from soda.
- HFCS (High Fructose Corn Syrup) is one of the most significant sources of calories in the average American diet.
- A breakfast-size container of Yoplait yogurt has more sugar than two Krispy Kreme donuts.

- A glass of orange juice has the same amount of sugar as a can of coke.
- There are 15 teaspoons of sugar in a can of soda. Would you put that much sugar in your morning cup of tea or coffee?

Here's a challenge for you:

Take the next four days and jot down how many grams of sugar is in every single thing you put in your mouth. Start by reading labels. Most sugar is hidden in processed foods, and we don't even realize we're eating it. If it doesn't have a label, Google it. You can easily find out how many grams of sugar are in most real-food items. I'm sure Siri or Alexa would be happy to assist you!

Next, just avoid pre-packaged, processed foods as much as possible. Drink water instead of soda. Use a tiny drizzle of organic raw local honey in your coffee or tea instead of a sugar-loaded coffee creamer. Plan your meals in advance to avoid the need for dining out. Choose real food and prepare it yourself. Let the sugar you *do* consume come from fresh fruit like an apple, berries, or a banana. Honey is also a source of sugar, however, there are numerous health benefits that come with consuming local, raw honey, namely a reduction in seasonal allergies. So, I give honey the okay, so long as it's a drizzle and not a teaspoon or two.

Make these small, simple changes gradually. The goal is not a short fast from sugar, nor do I want you to feel overwhelmed by change or deprived of anything you love. I'd rather see you take baby steps, changing one small habit or ingredient at a time so that you can create a new lifestyle that is healthy, enjoyable, and sustainable. I promise your body and your health will thank you in spades for giving it the opportunity to heal and not be so highly inflamed.

If you feel like your sugar addiction is too strong, and the cravings won't go away, check your meals to be sure each one is packed full of protein, healthy fats, and vegetables. This combination will help to stabilize your blood sugar levels and will go a long way in resolving sugar cravings.

Other steps you can take to bring those cravings to a halt:

- Get plenty of sleep. When you're tired, your body looks for a source of fuel to give it energy to keep going, so that's when sugar cravings begin.
- Quit the caffeine. Caffeine messes with hydration and blood sugar levels, resulting in cravings.
- Add sweet potatoes, beets, or carrots to your meal. They are naturally sweet and will satiate that sugar craving, but in a healthy way. You can also try eating half a banana or enjoy a small chunk off of a Green & Black's Organic Dark Chocolate Bar. The entire bar has only 12g of sugar, so taking a small chunk off of the end is virtually nothing and will quickly curb your craving while also making you feel like you've just splurged on something bad. It's not bad at all for you, though. Quite the contrary, it is highly recommended for a tiny daily treat of goodness!
- If you must cook or bake with sugar and you'd like to know of a healthy alternative, you can substitute any of these into your recipes. They are each natural sources of sugar, therefore, being less processed, but they should still be avoided or used in moderation as much as possible. Sugar is sugar is sugar – the body doesn't know the difference. It struggles to process all of it the same.

Barley Malt Syrup - It's made from soaking, sprouting, mashing, cooking and roasting barley, and it does move through the digestive system slower than refined sugars.

Honey - It contains enzymes, minerals, and vitamins. Local honey is good for building up your immunity to allergens in your particular geographical location.

Coconut Sugar - This is lower glycemic than regular sugar providing a more stable release of glucose into the blood.

Stevia - Use this one in limited amounts, and make sure it's 100% pure Stevia. It is very sweet and is a good choice for diabetics because it doesn't alter blood sugar levels.

Molasses - Choose blackstrap molasses as it's the most nutrient dense variety with a great source of iron, calcium, magnesium, and potassium in it.

SECRET #14

Lose that Unhealthy Excess Weight

Now that we've talked about what foods to eat, what foods to avoid, and the importance of crowding out sugar, it's a good time to bring up the importance of losing the unhealthy excess weight you may be carrying. To be your most confident self, and burn hot from within, we need to get you feeling comfortable in your own skin again.

According to the CDC, more than 93 million adults in the United States are obese. Seriously. Read that again. More than 93 million adults are obese in the US alone. That is crazy! This, of course, equates to billions of dollars being shoveled out to cover medical costs for obesity-related conditions such as heart disease, stroke, type 2 diabetes, and cancer.

If you fall into this category, don't feel bad. The good news is you hold the power to change the course of your health and your life. It all begins with deciding you've had enough, and that you want better for yourself and your loved ones.

Losing weight can often feel completely frustrating. You probably already know what you need to do to lose weight, but making those changes feels too overwhelming. You say to yourself, "Next Monday, I'm going on a diet." Then Monday comes and you do great! However, by the time the weekend rolls around you're ready to throw in the towel. You feel like it's just too difficult.

It's important to remember you didn't gain that extra weight overnight, and you won't lose it overnight either. I've said it before. There's no magic pill. However, there are some steps you can take to lose weight and keep it off.

To start, let's determine what your healthy weight should be. One method to determine this is to look at the Hamwi equation. This computation is based on inches and pounds. So according to this method, a 5-foot tall female would have a healthy weight of 100 pounds. For every inch that you are over 5 feet tall, add 5 pounds to determine your healthy weight.

Let's look at my weight as an example:

I am 5'2" tall. I currently weigh 129 pounds. According to the Hamwi equation, my healthy, ideal weight should be 100 + 5 + 5 = 110 pounds.

This would indicate I'm overweight. I assure you, I'm not. The problem with this equation is that it doesn't account for muscle mass, blood volume, or bone density. Other methods, such as calculating BMI (body mass index) don't factor those other things either. At least not accurately.

Have you ever noticed when you step on the scale every day the number can fluctuate 1-3 pounds from one day to the next? That's because your hormones fluctuate throughout your female cycle, your body holds onto water one day and expels it faster than usual the next, or you've been exercising, and your body composition is changing as a result.

What's the best way to determine your ideal weight? The best method, in my professional opinion, is to ask yourself, "How do I feel?" Also ask yourself, "Why do I think I need to lose weight?" And finally, "At what weight have I felt my best in the past?" The answers to these questions can speak a lot about your current state of health, both physically and mentally, and along with the Hamwi equation, can give you a target weight to set your goals for.

Overall, how do you feel?

- Are you lacking energy? When did you have the most energy?

- Do your clothes fit and look nice on you? What size do you feel best wearing?
- Are you confident and carefree when you're around other people?
- Are you easily short of breath when you exert yourself during a walk or some other low-intensity form of exercise?
- Are you embarrassed about how you look – to the point of preferring not to go anywhere or do anything that might put you in the spotlight?
- Are you thinking and focusing clearly throughout each day? When have you noticed you're most alert?
- What's your mood like? When has your mood been its best in the past?
- How well do you sleep at night? At what point in your life did you sleep best?
- Do the foods you eat agree with you, or are you experiencing a lot of digestive troubles? When did it all start?
- Are you suffering with a health problem, such as an autoimmune disease, diabetes, high cholesterol, high blood pressure, anxiety, irregular periods, or unusually horrible PMS?

How you answer these questions all factor in to whether or not you should lose weight. Do you see how the number on the scale doesn't actually determine your overall picture of health? It's only one way of looking at it.

If you want to lose weight, these are some best practices that will get you to your goal relatively quick and easy:

Drink more water.
I mentioned this earlier, but it's worth repeating. Drinking more water is one of the best habits you can get into that will improve your health, increase your energy, and help you to lose weight.

Add plenty of nutrient-dense foods to your diet.
You want to include a lot of healthy fats for adequate hormone

production and to keep you feeling satiated throughout the day. These include fats such as: avocado, coconut oil, grass-fed butter, ghee, nuts, and olive oil.

Before you question how adding fat (which is high in calories) to your diet will help you to lose weight, let me just say this. It's not fat that makes us fat. It's sugar! Sugar is what messes with our hormones, increases inflammation levels in our body, damages our gut lining, and when we consume too much of it, the over-burdened liver sends it out to fatty tissue elsewhere (tummy, hips, thighs, butt) to be stored.

Fat, on the other hand, provides a source of stable energy, it's good for hormones, and it satiates us so we aren't hungry as often.

You'll also want to eat lots of high-quality protein such as (organic, pastured, grass-fed, cage-free) meats, eggs, Greek yogurt, wild-caught salmon, quinoa, nuts, nut butter, and seeds. Protein is important for muscles, bones, cartilage, skin, and blood. You also use protein to make enzymes, hormones, and other body chemicals.

Finally, include complex carbohydrates for balanced blood sugar, energy, fiber, antioxidants, vitamins, and minerals. Good sources of complex carbohydrates are green vegetables, sweet potatoes, lentils, squash, bananas and other whole fruits, millet, buckwheat, amaranth, brown rice, and oats.

Manage your stress levels.
When you're stressed out, the body increases its production of stress hormones which will launch you into fat-storage mode. Why? Because your body doesn't know the difference between the stress you feel when you're being chased by a lion and the stress you feel from your financial situation. In either scenario, those stress hormones essentially shut down all other functions in the body in an effort to conserve energy and survive. Not something you want when you're trying to lose weight, right?

Stress also tends to result in emotional eating. Think of the foods you reach for when you're stressed out – sugar, processed foods, high calorie comfort foods. These all end up quickly converting to fat in your body.

One quick note: Don't confuse the fat in your body with the fats you eat. Fat does not turn to fat unless you eat far more calories than you can burn, in which case it gets stored in fat cells just like any other calorie source.

When stressed or under pressure, plan for success by having quick, easy to grab, healthy snacks nearby. If you like crunchy, which most people do, grab carrots, celery, mixed nuts, or an organic whole grain cracker with some thinly sliced cheese on top.

You can help manage stress levels by practicing stress reducing activities on a regular basis. Some ideas are a heart-pumping workout, yoga, an Epsom salt bath, reading a good book, listening to music, laughing with friends, and meditation or prayer.

Cook your food at home.
Home cooked meals are healthier because you have the power to control the ingredients and cooking methods, along with better control of portion sizes.

Watch your portion sizes.
The sad reality is we often eat way more food than we really need or are hungry for. Sometimes it's a social thing while kicking around with friends. Other times it's a stress thing while we're working through a problem. And sometimes it's a dining out thing where we are just given an enormous plate of food for one, but it looks like it's meant to feed the entire state of Pennsylvania!

Starting today, I want you to begin filling half your plate (relatively speaking) with vegetables which will naturally limit your grain and protein portion sizes, providing your body with plenty of fiber, antioxidants, vitamins and minerals.

When you dine out, split your entree with someone at your table or ask the server to bring half the portion already packaged in a to-go container.

Practice healthy socializing.
When hanging out with friends, practice awareness with how much you're eating. Rather than picking at finger foods, portion some of the food onto a plate and walk away. When you've enjoyed what's on the plate fully, then tell yourself, "Okay, I'm finished." You can still enjoy a glass of wine and conversation without eating beyond what you've allowed for yourself.

Chew your food.
There's something to be said for slowing down when we eat. It's hard to do when we're busy with career or raising children, but it makes a huge difference in how well we digest our food. It also helps with the signals our body receives around hunger and being satiated. Plus, you should take time to enjoy your food while you're eating it. So… slow down and chew your food really well. Wait twenty minutes before going for seconds. Once your brain catches up with your mouth, you may find you don't want seconds.

Exercise your body regularly.
Working out burns calories, improves mood, increases libido, increases energy, balances hormones, reduces stress, and helps to increase muscle mass, which in turn boosts metabolism and burns more fat because muscle burns more energy calories than fat. It also improves your endurance levels and strengthens the respiratory and cardiovascular systems. When you break a sweat, you're also eliminating excess endocrine-disrupting toxins.

To lose one pound of fat, you need to burn 3500 calories. So, if you're exercising six days per week, that means you need to exercise long enough during those workouts to burn around 585 calories or more. Tools like Fitbit or an Apple Watch can help you to see a clearer reading of your actual calorie burn throughout each workout. I also recommend logging your food, drink, and exercise into an app such as MyFitnessPal, because you can't change what you don't measure. Remember the S.M.A.R.T. method.

Finally, when it comes to exercise, to be successful, do what you love. Do it in a class or group setting, or meet with a personal trainer to get your workout in. The accountability, social aspect, and having it already scheduled makes showing up a lot more likely than if you try to go it alone.

Track your calories and sugar consumption.
Visit the URL below and calculate your maximum calories for each day based on how much weight you'd safely like to lose. If the daily calories are lower than 1200, then your minimum should be 1200. Sorry, but I really don't want your body going into starvation mode. When that happens, metabolism shuts down. I'd rather see you eat more calories and exercise harder than eat fewer calories. This is not a starvation program. Your body needs nourishment! (www.calculator.net/calorie-calculator.html)

You can track your calories and total grams of sugar consumed through MyFitnessPal or some other similar calorie tracking app. When it comes to sugar, it is suggested that women limit their sugar consumption to 24g or less per day and men hold theirs to 36g or less per day. This is from all sources, which includes natural sources like fruit as well.

Don't completely cut fruit out of your diet, though, because it's loaded with nutrients that your body needs. Instead, choose lower glycemic fruit like berries and pick only a few days out of the week to enjoy it. This allows for the health benefits while not over-indulging on it.

Invest in yourself.
Join the next session of The Better Body Challenge© or hire a health coach or a personal trainer that is knowledgeable in nutrition. Yes, it's a shameless plug.

The methods I share in this book work. They are the same methods I coach my clients through, and collectively over the past year alone I've witnessed more than 358 pounds of weight loss through my clients!

You can, of course, try to do this journey on your own and you may be wildly successful at it. Get a gym membership, grab a friend, and get started. Tackle your goals with a positive "no-quit, no excuses" attitude. Make a non-negotiable commitment to yourself. Work your ass off. It won't come easily, and it won't happen overnight. But if you set your mind to it, and you fuel your fire the way I'm teaching you here in this book, you'll have the body and the life you've always wanted!

Fuel Your Fire Action Steps:

1. Drink more water. Aim for 1/2 your body weight in ounces of water each day.
2. Get started with home cooking. Cook 90% of your meals.
3. Eat real, nutrient-dense foods. High protein, healthy fats, and veggies.
4. Supplement where needed.
5. Crowd out sugar.
6. Lose that unhealthy, excess weight.

PART 3

Add Heat to Your Body

Turn Up the Heat with Exercise

"I want my body like my coffee. Hot and strong."

– UNKNOWN

A while back, I saw news of a 90-year-old woman who completed a marathon. The video showed her running across the finish line with bright red lipstick on her lips and the biggest smile I've ever seen. I felt so inspired by watching her! She was thrilled and had to have been in great shape to be able to run that kind of distance and still be smiling at the end. She is no doubt a woman who is on fire for life!

It's clear to me that she had done things right with her body over the years. To be vibrant and full of energy at 90 years-old, she must have already known and mastered the secrets to living her healthiest life. To keep her fire burning hot, she certainly provided herself with adequate fuel, heat, and oxygen.

If a 90-year-old woman can conquer a marathon, you can definitely change your health for the better, don't you think? I always say health is a journey, not a destination. Even in your ninth decade of life, you will need to keep making good choices around food and fitness. That's what will keep your engine roaring.

Yes, your engine. Think of your body like it's this beautiful exotic car, and your insides are the engine. An engine gets hot during operation, which is normal. Well, you want your body to run hot, too. I'm not talking feverishly or hot-flashes kind of hot, but more like the good, sweaty, just knocked out the best workout kind of hot.

In this state of heat, you are more likely to feel truly happy, be healthy, and appear fitter. Your hormones will certainly function better, and your metabolism will work more efficiently. Your blood will circulate well, and your immune system will be better equipped to fight off foreign invaders. Your skin will be glowing. You'll produce a ton of energy. You'll smile more often, and your gut microbiome will be thriving!

Are you convinced yet as to why adding heat to your system is so important? So, there's a few ways to add heat to your body, through exercise, improved gut health, and improved hormone health.

Of course, heat will be generated through the action of exercise, so that's the first thing I want to talk about. When you exercise, your heart rate rises, and the blood begins to pump faster. This increased blood circulation sends oxygen to all of your organs allowing them to function optimally. It also gives your skin a beautiful glow while improving your memory at the same time.

Strength training or weight bearing exercise builds muscle. Muscle will turn your body into a fat-burning machine because it burns a much higher percentage of calories at a faster rate, and will continue to do so even during rest. Whereas body fat is much lower in calorie expenditure on a per-day basis. In other words, your metabolism fires up exponentially the more muscle you have.

The lower your metabolism, the lower your body temperature will be – usually below 97.8 degrees. People who are obese tend to run lower on body temperature. As steps are taken to increase body temperature, there is typically improved mood, energy levels, weight loss, and more.

Your muscles also make energy which results in the production of sweat. Sweat has a cleansing and detoxification effect, which helps to keep you healthy all the way around.

Not everyone loves exercise, but I definitely do. I love to feel strong and I love to see my body change with the different types of exercise I incorporate into my weekly workouts. I've been active my entire life. When I was little, I danced. Later on, I loved doing gymnastics. When I played with friends, there was often a trampoline involved. In high school, I ran track & field. When I was eighteen years old, I joined the military and flew to Fort Jackson, South Carolina, where I attended Army Boot Camp. That's where I developed a love for pushups, long hikes, running, and sit-ups. It's also where my self-discipline around fitness really blossomed.

After I had children, I trained with a personal trainer at the gym for six months straight and was in the best shape of my life. I also started running races. I ran a few 5k's and then a half marathon. I've done the Mudderella and the Muddy Princess. I've done a Spartan, too. I've been active in Kickboxing and Krav Maga. Follow me on Facebook or Instagram and you'll quickly see that I'm a strength training junkie as well.

That said, I haven't always been 100% active. There were years in-between where I wasn't consistently active at all, and I let many excuses get in the way. The problem for most people who avoid working out is they don't want to give up laziness for working up a sweat. They claim to hate exercise. It's not that the exercise sucks. It's that the sacrifice to go do it sucks. What they often discover is that once the workout is completed, there are no regrets. The sense of accomplishment and the feel-good hormones made it all worth it.

Exercise is so beneficial for your body, and it really should be one of your top priorities. Aside from improving your metabolism and helping you to lose weight, exercise is also a mood enhancer. It's good for clearing your mind of stress, improving your mood through those feel-good endorphins, and it helps to regulate hormones.

Exercise is also a confidence booster. Get yourself to the gym regularly and watch how your confidence begins to soar. Your clothes will begin to fit better, and your skin will glow. Your hair will shine, too. You'll look lean, muscular, and sexy as hell. If you're married or dating someone, this newfound body and confidence will be a perk to your relationship! You may find yourself flirting more with your lover and your sex drive will be out of this world.

When I feel good about myself, I speak with more boldness and confidence. I carry myself differently. I even walk differently! You will, too!

Exercise is also a healthy way to reduce stress. Being active is a far better choice for stress reduction than turning to self-destructive addictions. I really hate yoga. To me, it's dull. However, when I'm stressed out, I'll do a 30-minute yoga session because I know it will help relax me and get my breathing under control.

If I feel fueled with anger, I'll go for a run because I know running takes everything out of me. It burns off all of that negativity and leaves me filled with endorphins and a renewed attitude.

Exercise is the best way (along with healthy eating) to lose weight. There is no magic pill for weight loss. If you want to lose weight, you have to get up off the couch and move your body. You have to eat clean and reduce your portion sizes in the kitchen. You have to follow the suggestions in this book.

Exercise will improve your quality of life as you age. I don't know about you, but I don't want to feel older than I actually am. As we age, our body naturally slows down and just can't do the things we could do when we were twenty. But if we keep exercising and keep our body active, we'll age with so much more quality of life than if we just give up and sit in a chair all day. That 90-year-old marathon beauty must have felt decades younger than her true age!

I'm often asked what type of exercise is best and for how long. Many people avoid exercise because they don't know what they should be doing. Some are very out of shape and exercise takes a huge effort. Others have told me the thought of stepping foot inside a gym is terrifying. They're worried about people judging them. Working with a certified personal trainer can be a great benefit in all of these scenarios!

However, if you choose to take the fitness journey on your own, here are some of the best exercise options to go with:

Walking – simple, yet powerful. Anyone can do this regardless of fitness level.

Strength training – muscles not used will lose strength over time. The more muscle you have, the more calories you burn and the easier it is to get the body you want.

Tai Chi – this is a Chinese martial art that combines movement and relaxation that is good for body and mind. It's particularly useful for those looking to improve balance.

Swimming – this is a safe and effective way to challenge your body without the risk of injury to joints. It's also great for improving your mood.

Yoga – both strengthening and lengthening, yoga is excellent for keeping the body lean and limber. It's also really good at reducing stress and has been shown to immediately lower cortisol levels in the body.

Body conditioning – one of the best tools for getting fit is using your own body as the tool for fitness. Not only does this improve balance and stability, but it strengthens as well.

HIIT training – HIIT stands for High Intensity Interval Training. This is actually one of the best ways to exercise for weight loss. It is also recommended training for those who struggle with adrenal fatigue. These are workouts that get your heart rate elevated for short periods of time, such as two minutes, with a shorter interval, such as one minute, of a much lower heart rate.

I recommend mixing them up. In other words, don't just pick one and do only that activity. Do something different each day. Listen to your body. If you're feeling fragile or lacking coordination and focus, give kickboxing or martial arts a try. If you're extremely tense and stressed, go with more relaxing types of exercise like Pilates or Yoga.

In any fitness plan, fun should be the key. If you don't enjoy it, you won't stick with it, so find your passion in the workout, and you'll be set for life!

10 Reasons I Want You to Start Working Out Regularly

1. To achieve your fitness goals
2. For a stronger, more lean, and healthier body
3. For happy, healthy hormones
4. To be more alert, creative, and productive
5. For the mood and confidence boost
6. To increase your sex drive
7. To increase your energy levels
8. For the sexy AF muscles
9. To relieve stress
10. For the title of badass!

Target 420 minutes of exercise per week, or about an hour of exercise per day. This will significantly decrease your risk of premature death. Although health benefits kick in with as little as 30 minutes per day. I suggest you strive to do three days per week of Cardio, three days per week of Strength Training, and one day per week of Yoga, Tai Chi or PiYo (Pilates-Yoga combination).

So, for example, your workout week might look like this:

MONDAY: Cardio Kickboxing
TUESDAY: Strength Training – Upper Body
WEDNESDAY: 3 Mile Run
THURSDAY: Strength Training – Lower Body
FRIDAY: Zumba
SATURDAY: Strength Training – Body Conditioning/Core
SUNDAY: Tai Chi

What and When to Eat Before a Workout

Two common questions my clients ask is, "What should I eat prior to a workout, and when is the best time to eat?"

My answer is, it really depends on you and your body. Everyone's body and needs are different. Of course, fueling your body with quality nutrition and plenty of water consistently is a first step. Also, you need sleep, at least 7-9 hours per night.

Next, decide how hard your workout will be, and then fuel up accordingly. For high-intensity exercise, reach for carbs. Longer, less intense workouts, reach for healthy fats. For all workouts, include a protein source as it improves muscle protein synthesis and helps with recovery.

Ideally, it's best to eat a complete meal containing protein, carbs, and fat 2-3 hours before your workout. But I realize that's not always an option, especially if you're an early morning gym-goer. So, in that case, target eating 45-60 minutes before your workout and pick something easy to digest.

Here are a few great ideas for pre-workout meals if you are limited with time before a workout:

- A piece of fruit, like a banana.
- One or two homemade energy balls.
- A high-quality, all-natural nutrition or protein bar.
- Plain Greek yogurt and a chopped-up Granny Smith apple with a tiny bit of raw, local honey drizzled over the top. Add a sprinkle of cinnamon and a few chopped pecans.
- Protein smoothie made with milk, a high-quality protein powder, and a small serving of fruit.
- A cup of oatmeal topped with chopped nuts and 1/2 a banana.

Ultimately, you'll need to try a few different methods, listen to your body, and see what works best for you.

SECRET #16

Turn Up the Heat in Your Gut

"All disease begins in the gut."

– HIPPOCRATES

N ow that you've been working on adding fuel to your fire, let's heat things up even more, starting with the gut. Your gut is a big part of the engine in the exotic car that is your body. This engine is where digestion, metabolism, and absorption happen. The outcome of those processes then creates energy, or in other words, heat!

Your gut area is lined with more than 100 million nerve cells, and it is often referred to as your second brain. It actually talks to your brain via the vagus nerve, releasing hormones into the bloodstream. Once hormones are released, it only takes a few moments for them to send signals to your body. These signals communicate that you're hungry, tired, sad, aroused, or feeling awesome.

There have been studies directly connecting the state of our gut health to obesity, eating disorders, depression, autism, ADHD, anxiety, hormone balance or imbalance, chronic inflammation in the body, quality of sleep, energy levels, metabolism, skin health, autoimmune conditions, food allergies, and so much more.

So, you can imagine how important it is to have a durable, healthy, gut lining and diverse microbiome. The healthier the state of your gut is, the more heat you will be generating in your metabolism and mood, to name just a few ways of looking at it.

Fun Fact:

The total surface area of your gut is approximately the size of half a badminton court or the size of a small studio apartment!

The gut microbiome refers to the billions of live bacteria humans have in their gut, but it also includes things such as fungi and viruses. It has been estimated that there are approximately 35,000 different strains of bacteria within our body. Yet we attempt to avoid germs like they're the plague, no pun intended.

We regularly wash our hands, reach for the antibacterial wipes or soap, and we cringe when someone sneezes in our direction. The truth is we are like one big walking Petri dish of bacteria. According to various scientific studies, there are ten times more bacterial cells in your body than there are human cells. Gross, right? But it's actually a good thing.

It all begins the moment you're born as you take in a mouthful of bacteria on your way through the birth canal. This continues as you have human contact with your mother, your father, your pets, and other people around you.

Bacteria produce chemicals that help to equip us with energy and pull nutrients from our food. Intestinal bacteria influence the function of immune cells, as well. Taking a high-quality probiotic and eating naturally fermented foods such as yogurt, kimchi, kombucha, and sauerkraut are great ways to boost the good bacteria in your gut, therefore, boosting your immune system.

Taking good care of your gut health can make a huge difference in your overall physical health and happiness. The good news is it's not too hard to course-correct the state of your gut health. You've already started improving things by following the nutrition guidelines I shared earlier in this book.

Don't skip past this step for adding heat to your fire. A healthy gut will help you to enjoy happiness, and it will eliminate feelings of anxiety, too. It also helps with reducing circulating cortisol in the body, supports healthy aging, reduces your risk for obesity or being overweight, supports the production of short-chain fatty acids, which inhibit the growth of bad bacteria, increases your body's ability to absorb calcium and helps to reduce oxidative stress. Having a healthy gut will also lead to a healthy BMI (body mass index).

A gut that is in a state of damage eventually leads to autoimmune disease. One autoimmune disease often leads to another. That's because the root cause of the problem – an unhealthy gut – is rarely addressed.

Odds are, you have gut problems. If you walk into your doctor's office and ask about it, he or she may look at you like you're speaking some foreign language. But if you were to visit a functional medicine practitioner, he or she may refer to it knowledgeably as increased intestinal permeability.

If you're experiencing cravings for sugar or carbs, excessive fatigue, have chronic diarrhea, constipation, or gas you likely have leaky gut. Other symptoms are nutritional deficiencies, headaches, brain fog, memory loss, and arthritis or joint pain. Watch for mood imbalances such as anxiety and depression and skin issues like acne, rosacea, and eczema, as well.

Diet is probably the most significant contributor to leaky gut, but other things are factors as well. The main issues are foods, infections, toxins, and stress. Gluten is a major cause of leaky gut, too. It causes your gut cells to release a protein that can break apart the tight junctions in your intestinal lining.

The integrity of your gut lining can become compromised and break down if it's continually being exposed to irritants through your diet or environment. Having a chronically stressful lifestyle leads to a breakdown in gut health as well. Even brief periods of stress have been shown to alter the gut microbiota. This all leads to low-level inflammation and can result in health problems of all sorts.

Refined sugar and excess alcohol also damage the intestinal lining. Sometimes an infection such as candida overgrowth, intestinal parasites, and SIBO (small intestinal bacterial overgrowth that normally grow in other parts of the gut) are to blame. Toxins are another problem causing poor gut health. They come in all forms – NSAIDs (non-steroidal anti-inflammatory drugs such as ibuprofen or Motrin), steroids, antibiotics, acid-reducing drugs such as Prilosec, and Nexium, and environmental toxins like mercury, pesticides, and BPA from plastics. Stress is another massive contributor to leaky gut.

If you suspect you have gut issues, start with focusing on improving your diet and lifestyle. Eat real food, particularly clean protein sources, healthy fats, and a wide variety of organic vegetables. Experiment with eliminating inflammatory foods such as dairy, soy, gluten, refined sugar, corn, and conventionally raised meat.

1. Avoid synthetic drugs such as Motrin, Ibuprofen, steroids, antibiotics, acid-reducing drugs, and environmental toxins the best that you can. If you're sick and you need it, then you need it. Just focus on supporting and healing your gut along the way.

2. You can support and heal your gut by taking high-quality probiotics and digestive enzymes. Taking a probiotic supplement for 28 days at a time, 2-3 times per year helps to maintain a healthy gut microbiome. Cooking destroys the natural enzymes in food, so digestive enzymes go well with taking a probiotic. They help to break down food and improve the entire digestive process.

3. Bone broth is delicious and incredibly nourishing to your gut health and your gut lining. Consider making it homemade with leftover bones, or you can buy it pre-made from your local health food store. Some good brands to try are Epic Brands, Kettle & Fire, and Bonafide. Drink a hot mug of it daily. Or you can add it to soups or other dishes that require a liquid base.

4. Fermented foods are natural sources of probiotics. Good choices to reach for are kefir, tempeh, kimchi, yogurt, and

even pickles. I often tell my clients to enjoy one pickle a day. You can also eat refrigerated sauerkraut or other fermented veggies.

5. Eat lots of foods that contain prebiotic resistant starch. This will help to stimulate the good bacteria in your intestines and maintain a healthy balance of bacteria. Good sources to reach for are lentils, white beans, chickpeas, cooked plantains, and cooled potatoes (like from potato salad).

Your next step is to repair your gut by consuming essential nutrients like L-glutamine, aloe, licorice, slippery elm, and marshmallow root. Collagen is also an excellent supplement rich in amino acids that will seal the leaks by repairing damaged cells and building new tissue.

- Consider adding gelatin to your diet as well. Gelatin can be consumed alone, or you can add it to your bone broth.
- Collagen can be taken in supplement form, or you can purchase it in powder form and add it to your smoothies, coffee, or soups. I really like Marine Collagen from Truvani.com.
- Be sure to eat plenty of onions, apples, and leafy greens as these all help to repair the gut lining and can help with preventing histamine release in the case of allergies.
- When you're eating, slow down and chew your food thoroughly before swallowing. In nutrition school, it was recommended to chew 30 times before you swallow. I've tried this before and let me tell you, it's not easy to do because we're always in a hurry to get things done. But it is worth giving it a try to help improve digestion and reduce gas and bloating.
- Increase your fiber intake, too. Aim for between 35 and 45 grams of fiber per day and introduce it slowly to give your body a chance to adjust. Make sure you're drinking enough water, or this could cause some gastrointestinal upset. Easy ways to add additional fiber are with a tablespoon of chia or ground flaxseeds added to a smoothie.

- It's also a good idea to light up your digestive fires with some digestive bitters. Good ones to try are dandelion, fennel, ginger, beetroot, and peppermint.
- Get your body alkalized by starting each day off with a glass of warm water and fresh lemon or lime.

Now let's talk about your poop! Did you know your poop can tell you a lot about your health? I know it may seem embarrassing to discuss it, but healthy bowel movements are a vital part of a healthy life.

The Bristol Stool Chart shown here is the standard primary assessment tool that you can use to identify the general health of your bowel movements. According to this chart, stool is categorized into seven types, which range on a scale from severe constipation to severe diarrhea. The low end of the scale signifies very dry stool, as a result of sitting in the colon for weeks. On the high end of the spectrum is a stool that has too much water, as the result of moving through the body too quickly. A healthy bowel movement falls into the middle of this scale, at 3 or 4.

		BRISTOL STOOL CHART	
	Type 1	Separate hard lumps	SEVERE CONSTIPATION
	Type 2	Lumpy and sausage like	MILD CONSTIPATION
	Type 3	A sausage shape with cracks in the surface	NORMAL
	Type 4	Like a smooth, soft sausage or snake	NORMAL
	Type 5	Soft blobs with clear-cut edges	LACKING FIBRE
	Type 6	Mushy consistency with ragged edges	MILD DIARRHEA
	Type 7	Liquid consistency with no solid pieces	SEVERE DIARRHEA

It's also important to mention that the number of bowel movements you have in one day really depends on how much fiber and fluid you're consuming. It's different for everyone, but ideally, you should be eliminating after meals, or at the very least, once per day. If you aren't, try increasing the amount of water you're drinking and the amount of vegetables and healthy fats you're consuming.

SECRET #17

Turn Up the Heat in

Your Endocrine System

Gut health and hormone health are probably the two most significant factors in having a well-functioning body and mind. When thinking about how hormones help to add heat to your fire, consider the fact that balanced hormones keep your body temperature and your metabolism on point. They also help to keep your mind sharp, your sex drive burning hot, and your mood stable.

The endocrine system is so delicate that the smallest imbalance can spiral quickly into an enormous problem, and gut health goes hand-in-hand with hormone health. An unhealthy gut will almost always negatively impact hormones, and your hormones are messengers that help your body to function, so they're kind of a big deal.

Estrogen, progesterone, testosterone, adrenaline, and insulin, to name a few, affect many aspects of your health. They are secreted by various glands and organs in your body, such as the adrenals, ovaries, pituitary, thyroid, and testicles.

Common signs and symptoms of a hormone imbalance include:
- Fatigue
- Depression
- Anxiety
- Unexpected weight fluctuations

- Insomnia
- Poor sex drive
- Digestive issues
- Hair loss or thinning
- Infertility
- Irregular periods

Keeping your hormones healthy and balanced can sometimes be a tricky thing, especially for women. If you have an imbalance, you'll want to make sure your doctor is monitoring your health while you take a natural approach to an optimal hormone state. I suggest you look into a well-recommended Functional Medicine doctor. Hiring a health coach who understands nutrition, gut health, and hormones is also a great idea!

If you were to go to a conventional primary care physician or even a specialist complaining of a health concern that pointed to a hormonal imbalance, he or she would very likely put you on birth control pills, insulin injections, thyroid medication, or some other synthetic hormone replacement therapy. I'm personally not an advocate for the use of artificial hormones unless it's a severe situation needing immediate resolution. Some people do need support through thyroid medication or insulin shots where natural methods won't resolve those issues.

From a broad view, synthetic hormones may have benefits, but the adverse effects on the body, specifically the gut lining and microbiome is, in my opinion, not worth risking your health over. Some birth control pills have been linked to thyroid dysfunction.

Additionally, relying on synthetic hormone replacement rather than treating the root problem naturally does a few things. First, it will only mask your symptoms, not solve them. Second, it could make you become dependent on taking a synthetic drug for the rest of your life, which could put you at higher risk for serious side effects like reproductive issues, anxiety, cancer, stroke, osteoporosis, and more.

There are a few ways you can have your hormones tested.

- **Saliva testing** will measure your hormones at a cellular level. It measures estrogen, progesterone, testosterone, cortisol, and DHEA levels. Providing multiple samples at different times of the day can give your doctor a clearer picture of what is happening with your hormone balance.
- A **urine test** is one where you collect every drop of urine for a 24-hour period. It's the most thorough way to test because it's able to measure your hormones throughout an entire day.
- A **follicle-stimulating hormone test** is what is used to see where a woman is at in her perimenopause and menopausal years.
- **Blood tests** are another option. These measure total hormone levels. Saliva and urine don't.

Hormone imbalances are usually caused by multiple factors like diet, medical history, stress levels, genetics, and exposure to toxins. Other significant contributors are poor gut health, obesity, systemic inflammation from a poor diet, smoking, excessive drinking, extreme or chronic stress, and adrenal dysfunction, which upsets sex hormone balance. The excellent news is there are steps you can take, using a natural approach, to keep your hormones balanced and healthy.

First, crowd out the carbs. Replace them with a variety of healthy fats. Your body needs those healthy fats in order to create hormones. Healthy fats will also go a long way in reducing inflammation levels, boosting your metabolism, and promoting weight loss.

Reach for coconut oil, which you can use in your cooking. For a quick energy burst mix 1 tbsp. coconut oil with 1/2 tbsp. chia seeds and spread on whole-grain bread. It also makes a delicious creamer in your morning cup of coffee. There are countless ways coconut oil can be implemented in your day–to-.day diet and routine.

Avocados, wild-caught salmon, and grass-fed butter all have natural antibacterial and fat-burning effects. These fats lower inflammation and are heart-healthy, too.

Consider adding an adaptogen herb to your supplements. Adaptogen herbs like Rhodiola, ashwagandha, holy basil, and medicinal mushrooms have been shown to improve thyroid function, reduce anxiety and depression, lower cholesterol, stabilize blood sugar, and support adrenal functions.

- Holy Basil helps to regulate cortisol levels.
- Ashwagandha and Schisandra are very good at balancing hormones. It is beneficial to your thyroid function and can actually help you to reverse adrenal fatigue, which is something that occurs when you've been through extreme stress.
- Throw Maca into the mix and all three will be very helpful in improving sex drive, focus, energy levels, and anxiety. You can find high-quality versions of these in supplement and/or powder form on Thrive Market.

Deal with your emotional state. Your emotions have a more significant impact on your health than you may realize. In Traditional Chinese Medicine, it is said that fear causes disease in the reproductive organs, kidneys, and adrenals. Feelings of frustration or anger can cause disease in the liver, which would lead to an estrogen imbalance. Being a worrier can affect insulin levels.

You can deal with your emotions a little bit better by exercising regularly, taking time for yourself to sit quietly alone and journaling, or spending time in prayer.

Eat well! The food you eat has a high impact on your hormone balance. Hormones are made from the amino acids that come from protein, and from the fatty acids that come from fats. Using high-quality sources of proteins and super healthy fats will go a long way in supporting your body in creating better quality hormones. Aim to eat a lot of healthy fats, clean protein, organic fruit and vegetables, gluten-free grains, and sea vegetables.

Get enough sleep. Less than 7-8 hours of sleep can disturb your natural circadian rhythm and lead to a hormone imbalance. Your hormones work on a schedule. Cortisol is regulated at midnight, for example, so if you're only going to bed at 11, then you're never getting much of a break from that constant stress response in your body.

One other thing people don't think about is how the body responds to exposure to EMFs (electro-magnetic fields). EMFs are considered endocrine disruptors. I realize it's pretty damn impossible to eliminate all EMF exposure in today's world of technology. However, there are certain things you can do to help reduce your exposure.

This is important because the thyroid glands are particularly sensitive to EMFs. Additionally, the thyroid affects almost every cell in the body, so if it's out of balance, you're likely to be feeling pretty terrible.

- Turn off computers and cell phones when not needed.
- Switch off your wireless network and Bluetooth connections while you're sleeping at night.
- Avoid storing or charging your electronics in your bedroom at night. A central "family" charging station isn't necessarily a bad thing!
- Also, avoid exposure to microwave ovens.

Get rid of environmental toxins. Your environment can be one more thing that gets in the way of balanced hormones. It's best to avoid environmental toxins when possible. The worst culprits are poly-chlorinated and brominated chemicals, BPA, phthalates, and flame retardants. PCBs and flame retardants block iodine from doing its job, negatively impacting thyroid health. Many of these toxins are present in our drinking water and foods.

You can reduce your exposure to these toxins by:

- using a drinking water filter
- installing a high-quality home water filtration system
- avoiding plastics such as water bottles, food packaging, and BPA-coated receipts
- using only natural cosmetics, personal hygiene items, and cleaning supplies
- eating organic produce, grass-fed meats, and wild-caught fish

Avoid excessive alcohol consumption. Alcohol is another endocrine disruptor when consumed in excess. It's been shown to elevate estrogen levels and decrease progesterone in women. Alcohol consumption also leads to a host of symptoms such as belly fat, higher risk for hormonal cancers, worsened PMS, heavy periods, and delayed onset of menopause.

Check your bloodwork. Have your doctor order the necessary blood work to see if you have any vitamin or mineral deficiencies. Generally speaking, most women with hormone imbalance can benefit from the following supplements: B-complex, Zinc, Vitamin C, Vitamin D, Omega-3 fatty acid.

Get group support. Jumpstart your health and happiness by joining an online group coaching program such as The Better Body Challenge©. You'll have access to me for asking questions, and lots of nutritionally sound guidance, fitness inspiration, as well as gut and hormone health discussion.

Fuel Your Fire Action Steps:

1. Turn up the heat with exercise. Get your body moving!
2. Turn up the heat in your gut. Strive for a healthy and diverse microbiome!
3. Turn up the heat in your hormone health. Make sure those babies are balanced!

"*Since I began my journey with Rosann Cunningham and the #BetterBodyChallenge I've dropped my resting heart rate (from 86 bpm to 66 bpm.) It's interesting and motivating to be able to look back and see the progress. Really hoping this next week and a half to continue to keep pushing to reach another small personal goal in my pursuit of a bigger goal. It's not always easy and often I have to dig down deep and remember my "why!""*

CECELIA MIDBERRY

PART 4

Supply Oxygen

SECRET #18

Supply Oxygen Through Self-Care

"Oxygen feeds fire. Take a deep breath!"

– UNKNOWN

One year. That's how long it had been. I was in survival mode, and it was all work, no play. Being entirely alone, an entire nation away from my family, and going through a divorce shifted my focus to merely surviving. I had spent a decade of my life as a stay-at-home mom to my two daughters, and suddenly I was moving out of our home, filing for divorce, working out child custody details, and launching my brand-new health coaching business.

I honestly had no clue how I'd hang on through any of it. I just knew in the depths of my soul that *not* surviving – *not* thriving – was *not* an option! I worried that my business (something I am incredibly passionate about) wouldn't take off, and I'd have to go work in a job that I hated just to make ends meet. I felt more isolated than I'd ever felt in my entire life. So alone, in fact, that when I went to have my blood drawn for my yearly thyroid and CBC checks, I burst into tears when the woman at the hospital registration desk asked me who my emergency contact was and I didn't have a name to give her. Divorce sucks. You don't just lose a spouse. You lose an entire family and countless friends, too.

Because I was so worried about my business failing, I worked my ass off day and night creating coaching programs, working with clients, studying even more nutrition, learning hormone health, and reading everything about gut health so I could be an expert for their needs. That didn't feel like enough. I wanted to offer even more value. So, I studied to become certified as a personal trainer through the National Academy of Sports Medicine. After all, fitness is very much a part of my business, too.

Since I am the face and the brand of my business, it's part of my job to set an example for what it looks like to be happy, healthy, and fit. This meant I had to somehow figure out and find time for hitting the gym daily, cooking healthy meals (for a table of one), and having my life put together, or at least be on the right path for meeting my own personal goals and desires. I had to practice in my own life what I was preaching to my clients. Unfortunately, I was falling short on self-care, sleep, love, and sunshine.

I had spent hours working on sales and marketing, had put together seminars and workshops, and had participated in trade shows. I worked feverishly to develop content for and launch my first online group coaching program, The Better Body Challenge©. My customer base really started to grow. I gained more private coaching clients. I continued running sessions of The Better Body Challenge©, and word of mouth brought me even more new clients. Before I knew it, I had worked with ninety-three new clients in one year.

Whew! I was feeling it, too. I was tired, but I kept pushing forward knowing I still hadn't achieved the level of growth I wanted or needed. But then, unexpectedly and tragically, my mom died. It stopped me in my tracks. I was in shock. She was my best friend, the woman who raised me, who was stronger than any other woman I've ever known, and she was the one person I literally thought would live forever. She was way too stubborn for God to call her home anytime soon, or so I thought. The emotional stress of that loss was devastating and nearly broke me. I never had the opportunity to tell her I was writing this book – she would have been beaming!

When someone you love dies, the shoulda-coulda-woulda's come to the surface. I should have spent more time with my mom, especially not rushing her off the phone during that last phone call she made to me. I had a coaching session I was late for. I could have traveled back to Idaho to see her more often. It was costly, but there was no reason I couldn't have gone alone to save money. If I'd known the last hug I'd get from her was the summer of 2018, I would have never left her side to return back to Pennsylvania.

Regret is a bitch. Grief shines a light on what needs to change. All work and no play aren't healthy, and it doesn't bring joy. Family is everything. My children have watched me work nonstop for the last year. They've seen survival mode, and they've no doubt felt it every time they are with me. What they needed – what I needed – was life balance. All three of us needed some fun. I needed to find my smile again. I knew it was time to step back from work, breathe, and see what I had been missing out on.

I booked a trip to the beach for the girls and me to get away. Sixteen hours of round-trip driving in the car, three glorious days of sunshine, sea, and sand, numerous girl chats and giggles. I faced some fears during that trip, driving over the Bay Bridge and through some tunnels. Because I'm terrified of both, conquering those beasts made me feel like a total badass. My beautiful daughters cheered me on the entire time. It was a fabulous mother-daughter bonding adventure the three of us will never forget.

I also booked a trip to Vegas with a sweet friend of mine for a girl's weekend. We explored the Vegas strip, soaked up the sun at the MGM Grand pool, shopped until we dropped, drank plenty, and had girl talk for hours. It was unbelievably therapeutic for both of us. A revelation of sorts hit me on that trip. Even though it scared the shit out of me, I knew it was time to start dating again.

There was already this great guy I had been having casual conversations with for several months. He had asked me out twice and both times I blew him off. But, after eight months of slowly getting to know him, upon my return from Vegas, I finally agreed to go out on a date. This handsome, intelligent, funny, and very caring man quickly became what I now call my man distraction. He is by no means a bad distraction at all. In fact, he has turned my world upside down with so much adventure, joy, peace, and romance. Without even saying a word, his presence in my life has spoken volumes to me on the subjects of self-care, love, sunshine, life balance, and sleep. My inner fire burns hotter now than it ever has. Oxygen was the element I was missing all along, and this man who I have fallen madly, deeply in love with opened my eyes and my heart to precisely what I needed.

I don't know what your current state of oxygen is, but I'm betting you could use a little or a lot more than you currently have in your life. Don't wait for regret or grief to be the catalyst for change. There are no takebacks. Time doesn't reverse. What you need is within your reach. It's up to you to grab on tight and let it fuel your fire.

You can't pour from an empty cup.

'Selfish' isn't a dirty word.

Fit your own oxygen mask first so you're able to help someone else.

I love the sound of all of that self-care wisdom! When was the last time you put on your oxygen mask? I certainly hope you're familiar with the term self-care and that it is one of your non-negotiable's, because your body and mind literally depends on it.

Self-care is any kind of activity that we are intentional about doing to take care of our mental, emotional, and physical health. Basically, it's loving yourself as you would others. When you know you've been burning the candle at both ends, and your resources are running low, it's time to step back in to replenish yourself and your health. The last thing you need to have happen is total burnout, right? If you don't take care of yourself first, you are virtually no good to anyone in your life. Not your kids. Not your spouse. Not your employer. Not your clients.

When you aren't engaging in practices that make you feel physically and mentally well, you end up depleting yourself of confidence and self-esteem. It's about maintaining a stable relationship with yourself, first and foremost. The great news is self-care doesn't have to cost any money at all. You can implement small habits of self-care throughout your week.

For example, you could spend an hour alone doing something that is just for you, like reading your Bible or drinking a cup of tea while watching the sunrise. You could block off time to take an Epsom salt bath complete with a good book and a glass of wine.

I always like to suggest unplugging for a certain amount of time each day. This act alone has many mental health benefits, most notably improving the quality of your life because you'll be able to engage in a real-life relationship face-to-face the way the good Lord intended.

Writing in a journal while you eat breakfast can be a very therapeutic way to spend an hour. Or you could set the alarm on your phone and indulge in a twenty-minute power nap. Ahh, doesn't that sound refreshing? If you have a favorite television show or you enjoy watching a good movie, that can certainly be a form of self-care, too. Quieting the mind through meditation cultivates a greater appreciation of life. So, when time allows, get in the quiet zone.

It may seem odd but making better choices around personal hygiene can be a form of self-care, as well. One idea is to increase your circulation by scrubbing your entire body with a hot, damp washcloth every morning or evening. This would be separate from your regular shower or bath. Stand by your bathroom sink to do it. Or, if you have one, you can use a dry brush to brush your skin in upward motions toward your heart. A dry brush feels terrific! I don't recommend dry brushing right before bed, though. It can be quite stimulating, which isn't favorable to sleep.

Create space in your daily routine for these other mental health ideas:

Take time to prioritize daily objectives. Looking ahead at your schedule to see what must get done and what is less of a priority helps to eliminate stress and mind-chaos as you tackle the day ahead.

Cut back on internet use by half. Instead, use that time to do more productive activities such as exercise, learning a new skill, or enjoying a hobby.

Enjoy a little bit of time in nature. Ten to fifteen minutes is all you need to step outside, let the sun shine on your face, and breathe in fresh air.

Self-care is NOT turning to unhealthy coping mechanisms such as drug use, over-eating, or alcohol (although I do love to relax with a glass of red wine-keep it to a minimum). These activities may feel good in the moment, but it is not something that is recharging to the soul.

People who turn to self-care on a daily or weekly basis experience better productivity, a stronger immune system, improved self-esteem, reduced stress levels, better hormone and gut health, increased passion for hobbies and other areas of life, and have more of themselves to give to others.

I was just sharing with a friend not long ago that when I take a weekend off from working and allow myself to relax, rest, or play all weekend, I hit the ground running stronger and much more efficiently come Monday morning. It's because I've taken time to recharge for a few days. That recharge pours oxygen into my life which then helps to fuel my inner fire.

Self-care is something I love to enjoy for myself, but as I mentioned earlier, a year of living in survival mode offered minimal opportunity for it. That said, I still had one non-negotiable, and that was my evening Epsom salt bath. It didn't matter if I was just getting ready for bed at midnight, I would still draw a hot bath and pour in some Epsom salts for an hour-long soak. Truth be told, it's probably the only thing that kept my health from failing given the intense amount of stress I was experiencing. That, and staying on top of nutrition and fitness.

Please don't say that you don't have time to care for your own personal needs. Here's a hard fact – you *do* have time for self-care, just like I did and still do. Not having time is just a lie we tell ourselves. If you're not practicing self-care, it's because you are prioritizing other things above yourself. You are just as important as your kids, your spouse, your church, your job, your friends, or anything else that is chewing up the majority of your time.

There is no reason why you can't take control of your schedule and carve out an hour for yourself a few times a week. Honestly, as much time as most human's waste scrolling through social media that usually only causes feelings of inadequacy, there's no reason you can't set time aside daily to love yourself. Even if only for a few minutes.

The amount of time devoted to self-care is completely up to you, there's no right or wrong answer for how much is healthy. A good rule of thumb is to give yourself thirty minutes to an hour every day to do something of your choosing that is not related to work or parenting.

Supply Oxygen Through Sleep

Until I'm six feet under
Baby I don't need a bed
Gonna live while I'm alive
I'll sleep when I'm dead
'Til they roll me over
And lay my bones to rest
Gonna live while I'm alive
I'll sleep when I'm dead

– BON JOVI, *Keep the Faith*

Jon Bon Jovi sang the words in his classic song "I'll Sleep When I'm Dead", but it's a running joke I hear from clients all the time. "I don't need more than four hours of sleep." "I'll just sleep when I'm dead!" "I can't go to bed that early!" Yes, even I have spoken those words a time or two. But maintaining adequate amounts of quality sleep is essential to optimal health and well-being.

When you're asleep, critical activities occur. Your body is working to support healthy brain function and maintain physical health. It's actually repairing itself. Thanks to your natural circadian rhythms (a 24-hour internal clock), your body knows what time it is. Just like waiting for Santa to come visit, the repair process doesn't start until you are in a certain state of sleep. Once you get there, internal organs rest and recover. Tissue repair, muscle growth, and protein synthesis occurs. Blood supply to muscles increases, and energy is restored. Hormones that help to regulate appetite control, stress, growth, metabolism, and other bodily functions are released. Memory consolidation occurs, allowing for the formation and storage of new memories, which is essential for learning new information.

Sleep helps us to thrive by contributing to a healthy immune system as well as a properly functioning metabolism. Even one night of missed sleep can create a pre-diabetic state in an otherwise healthy person.

Sleep also helps maintain a healthy balance of the hormones that make you feel hungry (ghrelin) or full (leptin). When you don't get enough sleep, your level of ghrelin goes up, and your level of leptin goes down. This makes you feel hungrier than when you're well-rested, which means there's a greater chance for overeating and gaining weight.

Sleep helps to improve your quality of life. You'll have more energy to make better lifestyle choices around cooking, exercise, and self-care. You'll be much more alert, focused, and creative. Anxiety, irritability, mental exhaustion, and bad moods will all be much improved if not eliminated. Your sex drive will be on fire!

Conversely, not getting enough sleep can be detrimental to your health. During sleep deprivation, weight gain and chronic diseases become a greater risk. There is also a high risk for accidents and injuries.

Loss of sleep negatively impacts cortisol levels in the body. This can lead to adrenal fatigue, inability to lose weight and/or weight gain, increased anxiety, hair loss, digestive distress, thyroid imbalances, and low progesterone, which in turn creates estrogen dominance. Too much estrogen puts you at risk for hormonal cancers such as ovarian cancer, cervical cancer, and breast cancer.

Sleep requirements are different for everyone depending on your age and your own unique needs. Typically, those who are over the age of eighteen should be targeting seven to nine hours per night, and those younger than eighteen require much more sleep.

If falling asleep at night is difficult for you, I promise you proper nutrition will help! What and when you eat affects your body's natural ability to both energize and rest. The more varied and clean your diet is, the more nutrients you'll take in. Your body will be well-nourished, have high energy, and will not need to rely on stimulants to stay active. Timing your meals and the size of your meals can make a difference as well. Try to eat your largest meal for lunch and a lighter meal for dinner. This will help your body to be efficient during the natural nighttime repair process.

Other ways you can ensure restful sleep are to limit sugar and caffeine intake and crowd out late-night snacks with yoga, journaling, or intimacy with your spouse. I also suggest avoiding late-night beverages that will lead to middle of the night bathroom trips.

Getting a decent night of sleep depends on creating a peaceful bedroom. There are many ways to do this. For example, you can paint your walls a calming color, use an aromatherapy diffuser, or invest in a new mattress.

A few other natural sleep aids you can turn to are calcium from a glass of milk, with a small handful of mixed nuts, half a banana, or a small chunk of dark chocolate which is loaded with magnesium.

If you have obstacles preventing you from getting sleep, such as children, spouses, worries, busy-brain, anxiety, pets, or working a graveyard shift, be sure the right people know and understand what your sleep needs are. If you can work dayshift rather than nights, request it! For busy-brain, anxiety and worry, keep a notepad and pen on your nightstand. When you're awake and your mind is busy, jot down your thoughts, and spend time praying. It's really sad to admit this but when I'm trying to sleep at night, sometimes what helps me get to sleep is to start silently praying for everyone I know and love. I usually wake up the next morning recalling only getting through about two names on my very long list.

If your kids are keeping you awake in the middle of the night, try to find the root problem as to why they are awake in the first place and solve that. Magnesium spray applied to the bottoms of the feet can do wonders for helping the whole family sleep well. Ask your spouse for help, too. Finally, discuss with your children how important sleep is for all of you and, if they are old enough, ask them to stay quietly in their own bed reading or drawing until they are tired enough to get to sleep.

One note on this: If your children are consistently awake in the middle of the night, this is not natural for children. Check their diets and/or instill the Amish Hour in your household. One hour before bedtime, no electronics are used including TV, cell phones, iPads, computers, Alexa, video games, and all of it. Read, do a puzzle, play with the dog, or talk to each other!

Earlier I mentioned circadian rhythms, and it's worth diving into that subject a little bit. Based on your age and circadian rhythms, there is an optimal time for you to go to sleep, wake up, exercise, and eat.

Circadian rhythms are specific changes in the body (mental, psychological, and hormonal) that are controlled within a twenty-four-hour internal clock. Things like sunlight, darkness, and temperature all affect your circadian rhythms. And your circadian rhythms change as you get older.

In the mornings, upon signals sent to the brain from light exposure, body temperature increases, and you should produce higher levels of cortisol (unless your adrenals are burned out). Cortisol is produced in response to stress, but also in response to your natural circadian rhythm cycles. It gives us energy in the morning, and as levels decrease throughout the day, it helps us to slow down and prepare for rest at night.

As we get older, melatonin in our body begins to decrease as well, causing us to wake earlier. This change usually starts in our thirties.

There was a study done by Oxford University that showed ideal wakeup times as follows:

20s = 9:30am
30s = 8am

40s = 7:30am
50s = 7am
60s = 6:30am

Based on that, it's important to adjust your bedtime to ensure adequate sleep, between seven and nine hours. Your best time for doing work or mental activities because you'll be most alert and creative is two and a half to three hours after you wake up. The best time for exercise is four hours before bedtime when you're at peak strength and lung function. The best time for eating dinner is for most people between 6:30 and 8pm. And if you'll be enjoying any kind of alcohol, it should be at least four hours before bedtime when your liver is functioning at its peak.

SECRET #20

Supply Oxygen Through Sunshine

"Even the sun directs our gaze away from itself and to the life illuminated by it."

– UNKNOWN

Sometimes I wish we entered this life with a bag full of do-overs. Think about it. We all have those days, seasons, or phases of life we look back on through more mature eyes and think, "Wow, was I a real dummy!" Wouldn't it be nice to reach into your bag of do-overs and wipe your slate of dumb actions clean? If I could do that, I'd have a lot of slate-wiping to do, but one of the first things I'd do is go back in time to my teenage years and take the bottle of baby oil away from myself.

I was a girl who worshipped the sun almost daily, and I never used sunscreen. Instead, I lathered myself up in... gasp! baby oil. Don't judge. You know you did it too! Everyone did, didn't they? Maybe it was just an Idaho girl thing.

Naturally, I burned a time or two, but mostly I just looked like a teenage version of the Tropicana baby. I'm not a huge advocate for sunscreen unless it's homemade and therefore not loaded with a bunch of unnecessary chemicals, but I'm also not an advocate for baby oil sun-tanning any more! That dumb move is definitely not health-coach approved.

I have always lived in reasonably sunny locations. In Idaho, where I grew up, we enjoyed four seasons, however, even when the ground was blanketed with snow, the sky was bright blue, and the sun was shining the majority of the time. When I turned eighteen, I moved to Southern California and enjoyed nearly two decades of daily sunshine and seventy-degree weather. But then my family and I moved to Western Pennsylvania, and my sunshine-filled days came to an end.

It's not that the sun doesn't shine here. It does. It just can't seem to find its way through the cloud cover very often. It's either overcast, thunderstorms, raining cats and dogs, snowing, or partly cloudy about ninety percent of the time. Or so it seems. My sunshine deficiency could be clouding my ability to see things clearly. There's no doubt my mood is different here than it ever was when I lived in sunny states.

Sunshine significantly impacts our mood! There's a hormone we all produce called serotonin, and this hormone is highly associated with altering our mood from depressed and sad to feeling calm and focused. During the evening hours when it gets darker, our brain makes another hormone called melatonin, which helps us sleep. When we aren't getting outside, and into direct sunlight for more extended periods, our serotonin levels will drop, and that is how seasonal depression occurs.

Light therapy can be one way to conquer this issue during the winter months. Although I've never personally tried one, I'm told light therapy boxes can be helpful. Probably the best way to overcome seasonal depression is to get outside for a walk or socialize outdoors with friends during daylight hours. The light and the company will work together for a significant mood boost.

I think it's important to note that exercise is one of the best anti-depressants you can implement! It's also good to be intentional about scheduling time outdoors. My man distraction and I took my daughters to a local lake beach a handful of times this summer with the intent to soak up as much of the sun and fresh air as we could, while we could. Not only did it give us glowing, tan skin, something fun to do, and quality time together, but we also got the benefit of the natural Vitamin D boost.

If you live in an area where the sun rarely shows itself, it's wise to get tested for a Vitamin D deficiency. Odds are, you're deficient. In that case, a high-quality Vitamin D3 supplement can make a huge difference in how you feel throughout each season. Vitamin D is crucial for optimal hormone function, gut health, calcium absorption, and healthy bones. If you are obese or have dark-colored skin, you may be more susceptible to a deficiency and would, therefore, certainly benefit from supplementation.

Keep in mind that Vitamin D3 is a fat-soluble vitamin which means two things. One, you can get too much of it which can be dangerous. Always check with your doctor to be sure your Vitamin D level is where it should be. And second, fat-soluble vitamins should be consumed with a healthy fat to increase absorption. So, take it with a meal or get one that comes combined with fish oil, such as Nutritional Frontiers Omega 3D.

I personally love a bright sunny home. Whenever possible, I open all of the blinds and curtains letting all of that daylight and sunshine in. Seeing the sunlight through the windows adds energy to my step and a smile to my face. It also helps to keep the houseplants alive, which increases oxygen in the air. Another great way to boost sun exposure and mood is to open the windows when temperatures allow for it so the fresh outdoor air can get into your home. This also has a cleansing effect on your home during sick season.

When exposed to the sun's ultraviolet rays, your skin creates Vitamin D. However, you need to be directly exposed to the sun long enough for that to occur. This is especially true if you live in an area where there are fewer daylight hours. If skin cancer is a concern for you, definitely use sunscreen and cover up when you feel it's necessary. But keep in mind that it's said a moderate amount of sunlight can be cancer-preventative because of the precursor to Vitamin D produced by ultraviolet B rays. About 15-20 minutes, or when your skin begins to turn slightly pink, is sufficient, and you should expose large amounts of skin when you're sunbathing. If you plan to be out in the sun for extended periods of time, use a sunscreen and apply it *before* you go out.

A note on sunbathing: The sun's ultraviolet B (UVB) rays are what interacts with 7-dehydrocholesterol (7-DHC) to create Vitamin D, and UVBs are the strongest between 10am and 2pm. Outside of those hours, UVA is dominant. These are the rays that are more likely to damage DNA and produce sunburn. More is not always better when it comes to getting sun. As an alternative, if you want to get more beneficial rays, you can expose your arms for a while, then cover them up, then expose your legs or face, and so on.

Oddly, it's said that the sun can help to heal various skin disorders such as eczema, acne, and psoriasis. What many don't realize is that improving gut health will also clear those skin disorders up!

WHO (World Health Organization) agrees with getting between five and fifteen minutes of sunlight on your arms, hands, legs, and face a few times a week. This is enough to enjoy the vitamin D boosting benefits of the sun. However, for this to happen, the sun needs to be able to penetrate the skin. So, using sunscreen or wearing clothing over these areas will not provide the benefits of vitamin D because your body won't receive the rays to be able to make it.

To avoid hormone-disrupting chemicals, consider making your own homemade natural sunscreen. For moderate sun exposure, even just mixing something simple like coconut oil, shea butter, zinc oxide, and red raspberry seed oil can be an effective sunscreen without any dangerous chemicals. There are numerous sunscreen recipes online that you can find with a quick search on Google. I'm sure Siri or Alexa would be happy to assist you!

Bottom line: sunshine improves overall health and happiness, which is a much-needed source of oxygen for that inner fire of yours to burn hot. So, make it a priority to soak up some sunshine daily, if possible.

Supply Oxygen Through Love

"One day you will kiss a man you can't breathe without and find that breath is of little consequence."

– UNKNOWN

When you meet a great guy who lights up your smile, speaks your same language of badassery, loves to work out, eats healthy, cooks for you, stocks up on your favorite wine and dark chocolate, and takes you to the pistol range on a Sunday afternoon just for fun, you think to yourself, "Wow, he might be a keeper!"

Loneliness sucks. I know this because I lived it day in and day out for a year after I moved out of the home I'd lived in with my daughters and their dad. Most nights I would eat dinner alone. Every night I crawled into bed alone. I was all alone in figuring out the details of my business while also being the business product myself. My ex and I do co-parent very well, but the reality is in my home, I have had to parent alone. Every obstacle that surfaced, it was up to me to figure out the answer. When my mom passed away, I grieved and still do, alone. Add holidays to the list of lonely, too.

So, when I finally agreed to go on a date with the handsome guy I'm head over heels in love with and adoringly refer to as my man distraction, it was no surprise to me that I didn't want our date to end. I had craved this kind of human connection for so long. Casually texting with him for eight months hadn't been enough. I knew immediately that we needed another date and another. Our relationship was so strong, right from the start. I had no doubt that I was with the future love of my life.

Humans are not designed to do life alone. We all need and crave love and connection with other human beings. When we have love in our lives, there are immense benefits to our health and happiness. Not having the desire to mindlessly shove food in your mouth – just because – is one of those benefits. When you're in love, you're high on life. You feel consumed with passion. A major human need is being met, so food becomes an afterthought. When you do enjoy a meal, it's healthier because you care about how you look and feel. The desire to remain trim and attractive for your lover is strong.

A study by the Health and Human Services Department revealed that couples who are married have fewer doctor visits and shorter hospital stays. A happy, healthy relationship also equates to lower blood pressure and reduced instances of depression. The longer the relationship, the less anxiety one experiences. Long-term couples are less likely to complain of headaches or back pain. Not having to face life alone aids in stress management. People who are happy and in love experience more periods of calmness which strengthens the immune system and allows the body to heal faster, too. Loneliness is associated with all-cause mortality (dying for any reason). Married couples have a longer lifespan, mainly due to being deeply connected through love with another person.

Oxytocin, the love hormone, plays a massive role in how couples feel about each other and about their relationship. Dopamine, serotonin, and oxytocin are often referred to as our "happy hormones." They work together when you're attracted to another person. Your brain releases dopamine, your serotonin levels increase, and oxytocin is produced. What happens next is a surge of positive emotion. You may even feel an addiction to one another. Also seeing a picture of your lover can increase dopamine levels bringing intense pleasure. This carries over into the strength and the length of the relationship, which ultimately affects health and happiness, too. In 2012, researchers reported that people in the first stages of romantic attachment had higher levels of oxytocin, compared with non-attached single people. These levels continued for six months or longer.

When couples put forth a consistent effort to flirt with one another, remain positive in communication and attitude toward the relationship, engage in frequent intimate time together, and are affectionate with each other, oxytocin levels stay high, and the relationship grows more passionate. The more oxytocin there is throughout the relationship, the longer the love is likely to last. What this means is the more effort you both put into it, the hotter the love between you will be, and the relationship will continue to grow.

It makes me crazy when I see people let themselves go and then let the passion die down in their relationship. They somehow explain it away as a natural progression when you have children, or when you've been married for a long time. So, what? Because kids come into the picture, your spouse and your health is no longer significant? What happens when the kids have been raised and leave home? It will be you and your spouse again (assuming your marriage survives that long) and by that time your health may be a total wreck and you and your spouse may feel like strangers.

Maybe you can rekindle the chemistry. Except by now, there isn't much attraction. You've both let yourselves go as a result of no longer flirting, no longer being intimate, and no longer dating each other. You didn't make the love of your life a priority. Being married a long time should not be an excuse for letting the passion die. Health issues should not be an excuse for allowing the love to die. If anything, they should be motivation to find the root cause of the health concern so actionable steps can be taken to bring healing back into the body. The relationships and love in your life are a vital component to good health and rapid healing. They also add oxygen to your life, thereby, fueling your deep inner fire.

So, you see, having love in your life is what I call life nourishment. But it shouldn't be just mediocre love. Why wouldn't you want it to be passionate? Why wouldn't your significant other want that, too? It's not too late to fix things unless you're no longer in love or you've already checked out of the relationship in your mind and heart.

Vital components in a loving and passionate relationship are respect, affection, intimacy, honesty, adventure, companionship, and open communication. Check-in with your lover to see if you're doing your part to bring these components front and center in your relationship regularly, and be willing to communicate your own needs in those areas.

Respect that your partner is an individual with their own dreams, passions, desires, talents, hobbies, and quirks. If these were not a problem for you in the beginning, they shouldn't be a problem now. It's not okay to belittle one another for the things that make each of you uniquely who you are. If your lover's job is dangerous or it requires long hours or some other considerable sacrifice, griping about it isn't being respectful to the choice they've made. You should be showing your lover that you adore and respect everything about them, and they should be doing the same for you – just like in the beginning.

Affection and intimacy are a big deal in a healthy relationship. Flirting falls into this category as well. You should be holding hands, kissing, gazing at each other, snuggling, and falling asleep close in the same bed together. Keeping the passion burning hot through sexual intimacy is vital in maintaining a strong bond with one another. A relationship without sex is called a friendship. If libido is a problem, keep reading. I have some health-coach proven tips that will get both of you fired up again!

Honesty and open communication go hand-in-hand in a loving relationship. You should feel comfortable enough being honest with your lover about how you're feeling or what's on your mind. They should be actively listening and considerate of your feelings as you're sharing. You can be honest while still maintaining a respectful stance, so be careful not to let a moment of honestly turn into belittling or accusing the other of some wrongdoing. When dishonesty enters the relationship, it's likely not to last long.

Adventure is something I mention because with fun experiences comes passion, laughter, excitement, and new memories. Don't stop dating. Make the dates fun and exciting. Dinner and a movie once a month get old after fifteen years. Go out dancing or go rock-climbing together. Run in a Spartan with your lover. Go to the shooting range. Hop on the river in kayaks. Leave the kids with a family member or a sitter and escape for a lover's weekend. This is the part where you get to live life fully. You don't have to be on vacation to have fun!

Companionship would be the final piece of the puzzle that makes a relationship hot. Just knowing you're not doing life alone is so important. You don't have to spend every waking moment together. Being present in each other's lives, available when you're needed, and even doing simple things like checking in with each other throughout the day means a lot. A text message to say, "I love you." A phone call because you want to hear his voice. A shoulder massage while he's watching the game. A foot rub after a long day. A nap on the couch together on a Sunday afternoon.

This is not a complete list of factors that make a relationship last. I'm certainly no expert as I've made my own fair share of blunders, but these are the big ones that I've noticed and evaluated in my own relationships. I've talked with countless women who have discussed these very issues with me during our coaching sessions, too.

One of the most significant issues couples fight about is sex. Men often have a much higher sex drive than women do, and therefore want it more often. There doesn't have to be a mismatch in sex drive between the two of you, though. This is a topic I'm very familiar with from my hormone health training.

As Jerry Seinfeld said in one of my favorite quotes ever: "The basic conflict between men and women, sexually, is that men are like firemen. To men, sex is an emergency, and no matter what we're doing, we can be ready in two minutes. Women, on the other hand, are like fire. They're very exciting, but the conditions have to be exactly right for it to occur."

Part of my job as an Integrative Nutrition Health Coach is to cover a whole-body, whole-mind, whole-life approach to health and wellness. This means discussing topics that may not be too comfortable to talk about. After all, being healthy isn't just about the food you put into your body. It's also imperative that you are being nourished off the plate as well!

I've found in my health coaching practice that it's actually quite common for women to have a lackluster sex drive. The reason for this is often caused by the stresses of motherhood. Sometimes women are overwhelmed by working outside the home. But usually, low libido is from low self-confidence and having negative feelings about her body. It can also be from hormone imbalances related to birth control pill use and the changing stages of a woman's life as she enters her menopause years.

If you're nodding your head in agreement, don't worry! I'm going to share with you some simple ways you can kickstart your sex drive and start reaping the benefits immediately. Yes, I said benefits!

Did you know sex is actually perfect for your health?

- Regular exercise increases sex drive, and a good sex session can be a great cardio workout. It's a win-win.
- Orgasm triggers the release of estrogen, which improves hair and skin quality.
- Women who are more relaxed and calmer have changes in the level of their luteinizing hormones that control the menstrual cycle.
- There are actually studies that show contact with semen during intercourse can be similar to taking an antidepressant. (Men always love to hear how their semen is a solution of some sort for their lady!)

6 Steps to Kickstart Your Sex Drive

1. Get into a regular fitness routine.

Strength training and body conditioning workouts are best for this purpose. Exercise improves blood circulation, which increases the odds of being aroused. It also naturally increases testosterone levels in both men and women. Plus, as you begin to see positive changes in your physique, your confidence will improve, causing you to feel proud to show off that hot new body. Choose a style of exercise that you love to do or will look forward to because that's what will keep you going back for more. Just make sure that whatever you choose has a component of strength and/or conditioning work with it. Building muscle is critical here!

2. Eliminate stress or find ways to manage it.

Stress is a dangerous libido killer. Chronic stress directly impacts hormone balance and gut health. The result is systemic inflammation, weight gain, autoimmune disease, digestive issues, and a whole host of other aggravating symptoms that won't contribute to feelings of arousal or sexiness! A few natural ways to reduce stress are practicing yoga, meditating, or spending quiet time alone, exercising, journaling, and earthing.

3. Get lots of quality sleep.

Most people aren't getting adequate rest because their bedroom isn't a sanctuary for quality sleep to occur. Make sure you have a comfortable mattress and bedding. Turn the temperature down a bit cooler than usual before bed. You'll sleep much better in a more comfortable room than one that is too hot. Turn off the TV or anything else that emits light or noise during sleep hours. Diffuse essential oils such as lavender or ylang-ylang. Go to bed earlier to ensure a minimum of seven hours of sleep before your alarm goes off.

4. Eat foods high in antioxidants and phytonutrients.
These foods will naturally rev up your sexual engine. Good choices are oysters, figs, almonds, dark chocolate, and pomegranates.

- Oysters are rich in zinc which is necessary for testosterone production. They also have two rare amino acids: D-aspartic acid and N-methyl-D-aspartate, which increase sex hormone production.
- Figs contain an amino acid that increases the production of nitric oxide. This amino acid is necessary for expanding blood vessels and sending blood flow to those sensitive parts where sexual arousal occurs.
- Almonds reduce inflammation and improve circulation, which directly boosts sex drive and fertility.
- Dark chocolate is rich in magnesium and B vitamins, but it also contains a unique compound called phenylethylamine, which triggers the production of the same endorphins produced during sex.
- Pomegranates boost testosterone levels in both men and women, and they improve the quality of sperm.

5. Think about sex.
When we engage our thoughts with what we'd like to do, our body will follow. It's easy to spend all of our time thinking about our endless to-do list. Doing so prevents us from really getting in the mood or even enjoying sex when the opportunity arises. Don't be shy! It's okay to think about it! Think about what you know feels good or what you know has turned you on in the past. Then flirtatiously share those thoughts with your lover, even if only by email or text. You might as well let him know you're getting in the mood!

6. Do it. Frequently.
The more sex you have, the more your body will crave it. So even if you aren't feeling in the mood for it, take a deep breath and do it

anyway. This includes allowing for self-pleasure. No, it's not dirty. It's helpful to know your body and understand what pushes you over the edge! Over time, your body will thank you with a naturally increased desire!

Fuel Your Fire Action Steps:

1. Supply oxygen through self-care. Block out 30-60 minutes per day.
2. Supply oxygen through sleep. Aim for 7-9 hours per night.
3. Supply oxygen through sunshine. Schedule regular exposure to direct sunlight.
4. Supply oxygen through love. Nurture the love and intimacy in your life.

"I have been working with Rosann for a year and she has helped me to make so many positive life changes. She is great at teaching you what you need to do to be healthy but is also so supportive when you struggle to follow what she teaches you. She encourages you to keep trying and gives you props for the changes you make, whether it's big or small. I have loved working with and learning from Rosann. As she says, when you have Rosann as a health coach, you gain both a health coach and a friend, all in one. You won't regret meeting with Rosann and learning more about what she can do for you and your health!!"

–NICOLE MATHIESON

PART 5

Let Your Fire Burn Hot

SECRET #22

Keep a Positive "No-Quit" Mindset

"There's no need to wait for the bad things and bullshit to be over. Change now. Love now. Live now. Don't wait for people to give you permission to live, because they won't."

— KRIS CARR

You did it! You've fueled your inner fire, and now it's time to really let it burn hot. Those who succeed in achieving their dreams have one thing in common. They never give up. Having a strong burning fire within is like having an energy force that so fiercely and passionately exclaims, "I will not quit!" Your inner fire is what will motivate you to get out of bed every morning and chase after the life and the dreams you want to see happen. It's so important that you keep your fire burning hot.

As I mentioned at the beginning of this book, life isn't always rainbows and unicorns. You're gonna have days that downright suck. You may even fall off the wagon a time or two. Let's hope just briefly! You've come this far, and I hate to see you backslide. Everything I've taught you up to this point is a lifestyle. It's not a diet or an idea. If you stick with it, it will become just the new norm for you. Call it your best way of living. Stick with it, and you'll look and feel incredible! Right now, the momentum is going, so let's talk about what you need to do to keep it at full throttle.

Adopt a positive, no-quit mindset. Having a positive attitude creates a happy life. It also helps you to live a goal-oriented life. When you're chasing down goals and making big accomplishments, your confidence will be out of this world. Plus, it'll naturally attract more positive energy from the world around you. This means you may have to change your thinking. There's a great quote by Henry Ford. "Whether you think you can, or you think you can't, you're right."

Be persistent. Persistence fits the mold for a no-quit attitude.

Be consistent. Consistency and passion will push you to accomplish anything you set your mind to.

Those are the habits and the mindset I've had, and it keeps me on course for the happy, healthy, and fit lifestyle I know is best for me. It's not always easy to stay motivated and disciplined to exercise or eat the right foods. Some days I really struggle to push forward towards my goals. I still have emotionally hard days trudging through divorce details and grieving the loss of my mother.

When this happens, I try to focus on doing good in my world. It feels good to give generously of myself and my resources. I attempt to live each day happily. Instead of focusing on the problem that has me wanting to give up, I focus on the possible solutions.

Music has been a lifesaver for me when it comes to mood regulation. A good song can really change my attitude and outlook. Laughter can do the same thing. I can't tell you how many times I've been in a funk and logged into Facebook to see some ridiculously funny meme flash across my newsfeed causing me to literally bust out laughing. Whatever it takes to get a giggle in, right?

Not gonna lie, though. There have been plenty of mornings where I wanted to stay in bed with the covers pulled over my head. I've had countless evenings of dining alone where the temptation to have a bowl of cereal for dinner was hard to resist. There have been plenty of days where going to the gym alone to work out on exercise machines felt so unappealing, especially when there are other types of exercise I would much prefer to do.

What has kept me going is remembering what I want and how bad I want it. I am always visualizing the life, the health, the body, the career, the success, and the happiness I want. Having a clear picture of what I want and a no-bullshit, fearless attitude about it is what keeps me going. That's how I've stayed motivated. I always know what I want, and I want it bad enough to work for it!

It won't always be easy for you either. If it were easy, everyone would be living this lifestyle. There would be no sickness or disease. Obesity wouldn't be a thing. Relationships would never fall apart. Unfortunately, that's not our reality.

If the temptation to quit is brewing within you, I say this. Stop quitting on yourself. You are worth more than that! Pull yourself up by the bootstraps and figure it the fuck out! I've given you the tools, but it's up to you to put them to work. You'll have to work hard and be very intentional every single day, but it will eventually just become a part of who you are. It will all come naturally to you. When you feel defeated and want to give up, don't. The choice is yours to either be frustrated and quit or let the frustration fuel determination. The effort to be frustrated or determined is the same.

If life knocks you down, and at some point, it will. Stand back up, smile, and very politely say, "You hit like a bitch." Persist when things get tough! Don't ever settle for defeat. Either find a way or make one. Get creative! Think outside of the box. Every problem has a solution, and you can find one.

Look at how far you've already come. Celebrate your progress. Every day you gain more knowledge and wisdom about what works for you and what doesn't, which means you're getting stronger and wiser. Remember that setbacks are temporary. You can do this lifestyle, and you can do it well. Figure it out. As Marie Forleo says, "Everything is figure-outable."

I have had some pretty crazy thoughts go through my head in recent years.

"I think I'll go to nutrition school." — Check.

"I think I'll start my own nutrition coaching business." — Check.

"I think I'll start life over at 45-years-old." — Check.

"I think I'll get certified as a personal trainer." — Check.

"I think I'll write a health & wellness book." — Check.

"I think I'll run a Spartan. Maybe my man distraction will join me." — Check.

"I think I'll go back to school for my degree in _____. — Stay tuned!

"I think I'll open my own women's gym." — Stay tuned!

...and the list of "crazy" goes on in my head.

The goals I've already accomplished were scary and hard. Those I'm still working on? Scary and hard. Inner fire has been the secret to my success. Despite fear, I took action anyway. I've experienced so much growth my entire life, but especially in the past six years.

My no-quit attitude has helped me to be fearless. I am determined to work my ass off until I achieve what I've set my mind to. I enjoy the hell out of putting a checkmark next to all of it.

Why?

Why the hell not?!

Listen. If I can do all of that, alone and scared out of my mind, I know you can do anything your heart desires. All you have to do is keep that inner fire burning hot, adopt a no-quit mindset, and figure it the fuck out. You've got this!

SECRET #23

Be Authentically and Unapologetically YOU!

"To live is the rarest thing in the world. Most people just exist."
– OSCAR WILDE

When I started my journey with the Institute for Integrative Nutrition®, I felt like I was going to burst with eagerness to share everything I was learning with anyone who would listen. Health and wellness is my passion! It's not everyone's passion, though.

Sometimes my sharing was met with an eye-roll, skepticism, or awkward silence. This would cause me to feel discouraged. Doubt and fear would then consume me. I started to second guess if this was the path I should be pursuing. There are many days, even now as a graduate and business owner, where I feel like I'm a salmon swimming upstream. Not everyone is sold on the power of nutrition, especially from a holistic point of view. Still, I love what I've learned, it's common sense to me, and I've experienced excellent results in my own life and have witnessed it in countless other lives as I've grown my practice.

It's hard to fit out! It's hard to feel encouraged when family or friends aren't supportive of what you're doing. Here's what I've learned in all of this, though. You have to be authentically and unapologetically YOU! Let go of the mindset that places boundaries on what you are capable of achieving. Let go of the mindset that gives other people authority over your worth, your life, your choices, your future, your success, or your failures.

Be your own person – fearlessly and boldly. You get to choose to be authentically YOU, and you should never feel wrong about that, or like the real you isn't good enough to be presented to the world.

I don't know about you, but I want to live in freedom. If I (or we) continue to listen to negativity from the community around us, we will never experience true freedom, real success, or pure joy. Instead, we will live with failure, doubt, fear, guilt, and a lack of confidence. Who wants a life like that?!

You *can* be authentically you, and here's how:

Choose your friends wisely. If your current friends aren't supportive, genuine, loving friends who cheer you on when you're running toward your goals, or if they aren't there to pick you up and hug you when you fall, they don't need a front-row seat in your life. You can still be friends, of course, but it's not a friendship that you need to put a lot of extra time, heart, and energy into nurturing. It's okay to distance yourself a bit, and you shouldn't feel guilty for doing so.

Network with those who have similar interests. Not everyone will love what you love. That's okay. Find groups of people who have similar interests and pursuits and network with them on occasion. These are people you can bounce ideas off of, share your hobby or career excitement with, and learn from. Call it a mastermind group. You can find these groups by searching Linked In and Facebook, as a starting point.

Always, unapologetically, be yourself. Freedom starts with being yourself. Don't be a jerk, but don't be shy about who you are, what you love, or why you believe the way you do. There is nothing wrong with expressing yourself! Don't worry about what other people will think. You don't need to impress anyone. You don't need to gain approval from anyone. You don't need to walk on eggshells around people. If someone decides they don't like the real you, they will eventually move on, and that is better for you in the long run.

Don't set limits on what you're capable of. There are no limits to what you can do when you place your mind to a particular goal. Refuse to listen to negativity from other people or from your own fears and doubts. You are God's child! You are amazing and very capable! Chase after the passions He places in your heart. Trust that He planted that seed and has grown it for such a time as this. Go out and show the world just how hot your inner fire burns for the things you are most passionate about. You never know who you'll inspire or how many lives you may change for the better simply because you chose to let your fire be seen.

Have an Attitude of Gratitude

Expressing thankfulness in life is an excellent inner-fire habit to form. There is always something to be thankful for, even during those hard moments when life slams you face down on the ground. Gratitude is particularly helpful in maintaining a positive outlook on life. After all, you don't want to be the negative, toxic person in your circle. You know the one I'm talking about. The person who always complains or gripes about this, that, or the other. Living with constant negativity is no way to live. Neither is stepping into the role of a victim all the time. Find your inner badass and deal with whatever it is that's got you down. Look for things you're grateful for to help lift your mood and bring your joy back to the surface.

New York Times best-selling author Lewis Howes wrote a book called *The School of Greatness*. In it, he says, "Life is better when you develop an attitude of gratitude." So, what is an attitude of gratitude? In short, it's expressing appreciation and thankfulness for everything in your life and doing so habitually. Make it a daily practice to look for and communicate through words, pictures, or writing at least three new things you can be grateful for. Howe goes on to say, "if you concentrate on what you have, you'll always have more. If you concentrate on what you don't have, you'll never have enough."

I realize it's not always easy to find things you're thankful for, especially if you're feeling trapped in a hard situation. Tony

Robbins shared in his book, *Awaken the Giant From Within*, that when it's tough to come up with something you're thankful for, you can ask yourself the question, "What could I be grateful for?", and see if some ideas start to flow. Often the greatest blessings we have are right before our eyes. We just need to acknowledge them!

I'm a huge advocate for journaling, so my suggestion is to buy a beautiful journal to keep in your nightstand drawer. First thing in the morning when you wake, before you roll out of bed, grab your journal and do a 15-minute brain dump. You'd be surprised what will come out of your head and onto paper first thing in the morning! My most creative writing time happens at 4:30am when my alarm goes off.

If you're active in your faith, practicing daily prayer and meditation can be other ways of expressing gratitude and staying tuned in to what you have to be thankful for.

One final thought I have on this subject is this: speak words of love and appreciation to the people in your life that you care about. Everyone needs to hear the words, "Thank you," "I love you," and "I appreciate everything you do for me."

SECRET #25

Stay Focused and Productive

"**W**ow! *Look at you, all dressed up with makeup and your hair fixed!!*" It was the next morning greeting I received from the ladies at a retreat I had participated in. As I poured some orange juice and glanced around the kitchen, I noticed I was indeed the only one in the rustic cabin filled with twelve women who had gotten dressed, fixed her hair, and put on makeup. Not that it was a bad thing that the others hadn't done that yet! I guess I was just surprised to see I was the only one who had.

Given that we were on a restful get-away, I should have felt okay rolling out of bed, wiggling into a pair of jeans, brushing my teeth, throwing my hair back in a classic ponytail and calling it a day. I certainly didn't need to impress anyone. It seems the other women had the right idea.

But what about when you're not on a relaxing retreat? What about the time spent in the everyday trenches of motherhood, homemaking, or just hanging around the house? What if you work from home? Do we really need to "get all dressed up" for those days?

You bet your ass we do! Starting the day out with a shower, a decent looking outfit, makeup applied, and hair styled is essential in setting our mindset for productivity. When I get a shower, I feel clean and energized. I feel like I've had a healthy dose of much needed personal time, too! When I dress myself in a favorite pair of jeans, a pretty top, some cute looking accessories from my jewelry box, and cover my feet with a pair of shoes (slippers do not count as shoes), I feel confident and ready to tackle the day.

When I take time out to apply some blush, eyeshadow, and lipstick, and then add some curls to my hair, I feel sexy and fabulous! If someone comes over unexpectedly, I won't feel the need to apologize for how I look. If I have to run out to the store, I'm ready. 1, 2, 3, Go! No looking in the mirror wondering if I should put a baseball cap over my tangled mane or change into a different pair of sweatpants. No secretly hoping I don't run into anyone I know – which of course *always* happens!

When I'm feeling gorgeous and put together, my man distraction takes notice. I communicate in a more loving (and flirtatious) manner, I greet him with a smile and a kiss, and there's definitely a sense of passion "in the air" between us when we're together in a room.

Probably the most significant difference noticeable to me when I start my day out dressed and ready versus lazing in my sweats, is that I move faster, and I'm focused. I get so much more accomplished! Don't you?

I know it's hard to get focused and stay that way. The struggle is real for me too. There are plenty of distractions that pull me away from the work I need to do. Let's take workouts, for example. I can quickly come up with a million excuses for why I don't have time to hit the gym. Same thing with cooking a healthy meal. I still do it ninety percent of the time.

You and I have the same number of hours in a week. I have kids, too, and yes, they have active social lives and busy sports calendars. I work more than sixty hours a week serving my clients and growing my business. I have a home to manage as well. I cook and clean and also make time for a personal life. It's not easy at all. But it's important to me, and that's why it gets done. I'm nothing special. Human, just like you. And I'm definitely not always perfect at this. What I am is determined, committed, and passionate about living my healthiest life, not just for me, but for those who love me and need me to be my best self.

If you're finding it tough to get focused or to be productive, try stepping away from whatever task is at hand that you need to accomplish. Go for a walk or take a quick power nap. Sometimes a change of pace is all that's required in order to tackle it with a fresh mind and attitude.

We all have that ugly frog on our task list that we can't seem to get rid of. That's the one thing that should be a priority. You will grow in energy and confidence if you knock that one off the list today. Brian Tracy, author of *Eat That Frog*, says that your frog is your most significant, most important task, the one you are most likely to procrastinate on. For some people, their frog is a trip to the gym. Other people may feel their frog is a home improvement project. My frog was writing this book! It will change depending on the season of life you're in and what you're hoping to achieve.

To stay productive and healthy, set daily goals that will help get you one step closer to the life and the body you want. Break big goals down into smaller steps and schedule them on your calendar. Give yourself a deadline and stick to it. Resist the temptation to waste precious time scrolling through social media, watching the news, or laying around in bed all morning. Check your inner fire to see how hot it's burning. If it's down to a low smolder, quickly get yourself back on track with adequate fuel, heat, and oxygen.

Then get yourself up. Get dressed. Kick some ass. And repeat.

Do Something that Will Help You to Grow

Personal growth is the process of developing yourself to achieve your fullest potential. It's crucial for your maturity, success, and happiness, and it's the foundation of your health. When you take steps to develop and grow as a person, it affects every single piece of your life. Feeling more passionate about life is one significant benefit. Learning builds confidence. The excitement will spur you on to desire more growth.

A friend of mine used to be very shy. She didn't want to be in the spotlight at all for fear she'd be judged. I encouraged her to start small, step out of her comfort zone here and there. She did. Then I started talking with her about her passions and talents. I encouraged her to consider starting her own business. She did. With these small and then more significant steps, her confidence grew. She then signed up to get certified as a yoga instructor. Despite still having a fear of being judged, she leaped into her training, and she grew even more. Now she's opening her own place of business, teaching yoga classes. During our most recent discussion, she was sharing that she's ready to grow more. She wants to learn something new, take things to another level. This is what learning does for our confidence and our passion. It helps the fire within to burn unbelievably hot!

I say it all the time – life is not meant to be lived stagnant. You should always be striving to grow in character, in faith, in knowledge, and in wisdom. To do so requires being open-minded and stepping outside of your comfort zone to live a little, experience life, learn something new, and yes, even to make mistakes. Nobody is perfect. If you stay within the safety of the proverbial bubble that is surrounding you, you'll never grow, and you'll miss out on so much.

I have many chapters in my own life that I wish I could just rip the page out or scribble through the parts of my story that were painful or that I'm not proud of. The truth is those experiences made me who I am today, and without the life lessons and personal growth that came from them, I'd still be living those chapters rather than having moved on from them. With each new chapter of life, my legacy becomes more vibrant and full.

What are some ways you can stretch yourself to become better today than you were yesterday? I suspect there's already something on your heart that you'd like to do but have some reason for not pursuing it. What do you have to lose in trying? Your life is your story. Make it a good one!

SECRET #27

Develop a Strong Tribe

Humans are social creatures, and we're wired to connect. Meaningful interactions build deeper connections with the people in your life. Honest and open relationships feed your soul. But we live in an age where connecting face to face isn't an easy task. Many of us spend a lot of time in front of our computers or smartphones and very little time socializing in person. We need each other, though. We need a shoulder to cry on or a friendly ear to listen. We need people to bounce our ideas off of and those to cheer us on when we're doing something hard and scary.

It's said that you become the five people you spend the most time with. I have found that to be true in a lot of folks, myself included! So, take a close look in the mirror and at those around you. What do you see?

Are you...

- Your best self right now?
- Making good choices?
- Eating foods that are good for you?
- Exercising regularly?
- Physically in shape?
- Full of energy?
- Confident?

- Putting quality time with the people you love as a priority?
- Practicing gratitude?
- Giving the love of your life your best self?
- Smiling and laughing?
- Waking up every morning on fire for life?
- Full of determination?
- Optimistic and encouraging?
- Helping others?
- Active in your faith?
- Creating an outstanding legacy?
- Productive and using your time well?
- Being wise with your money?
- Taking courageous action?
- Challenging yourself?
- Being a good friend?

If the answer is no, it may be time to change up your circle. You don't have to altogether remove people from your life but be intentional about regularly surrounding yourself with those who will motivate you, encourage you, and inspire you to be your best self! It can make all the difference in your health and happiness!

In the Better Body Challenge©, my participants often renew for each session because they've come to know one another and support each other on the journey to better health. They're all in the trenches together going through the same stuff. They can relate to one another. They are a part of each other's tribe. They are also a part of my tribe!

The best way to develop your tribe is to start by getting involved in things that are important to you and what you're passionate about. If you love hiking, get involved in group hiking events and Facebook groups where you can connect with other people who share the same passion. If you love food and wine, sign up for a wine tasting event in your area and get social with the people who also show up.

View everyone you meet with gratitude. Be genuinely thankful for who they are as a person, and that they've come into your life.

Do your best to be on good terms with the people in your circle. Ask yourself if the issue at hand is really worth the fight. Most things are not worth fighting over.

Beware of people who become a part of your tribe but don't have your best interest in mind. They're with you, but they aren't cheering for you. Instead, they're waiting for you to fall flat on your face so they can say, "I told you so." If someone in your tribe is continuously complaining or tearing others down, distance yourself, or cut off the relationship. It's toxic and not one that will be good for you.

You can't have a tribe without giving them any of your time or love. That means you need to be willing to check in on them, listen to them, send encouragement their way, and cheer them on too. It's not all about you. They need you just as much as you need them. So, schedule time to interact with your tribe. Do some fun group events together or invite them over for a meal.

The beautiful thing about having a tribe is that you don't always have to be perfect or strong. When life happens, they step up and pour love your way. You're never alone when you have a tribe.

Fuel Your Fire Action Steps:

1. Keep a positive "no-quit" mindset. Be positive, persistent, consistent, and believe in yourself.
2. Be authentically and unapologetically YOU. Go out and show the world how hot your fire is burning.
3. Have an attitude of gratitude. Every day ask yourself what you can be grateful for.
4. Stay focused and productive. Eat that frog!
5. Do something that will help you to grow. Step out of the comfort zone.
6. Develop a strong tribe. Nurture the relationships you have with those who support you.

"Rosann is very knowledgeable and knows how to steer others into better health. She doesn't only focus on weight loss or fat loss but also on healthier eating, emotional and spiritual health, and all of the other factors that play into a person's overall wellbeing. This helps you not only lose weight but become healthier from the inside as well."

– CHRISTINA KUHN

PART 6

Watch Out for Fire Extinguishers

Laziness and Lack of Motivation

You've worked so hard this far to get your inner fire burning hot. The sky is the limit with what you are capable of achieving. You have total control of your health and happiness right this moment. You didn't come this far to only come this far. Keep pushing forward with your goals. Don't get lazy or complacent. The body forgets really quickly, so the slightest backslide can be detrimental to the results you've worked so hard for.

Being on a health journey has its challenges – for everyone! Every decision requires some self-discipline, right? Whether you work with me as your health coach or not, here's the thing: the excuses have to stop! Our human nature has given us the ability to come up with a reason for anything!

Here are some of the excuses I hear frequently (and have admittedly used myself!):

"I've been too busy."

"Life is just crazy right now."

"I don't have time to... eat clean, exercise, cook, plan, or fill-in-the-blank."

"Money is really tight right now."

"This week is shot; I'll just start next week."

"One day I'd like to, but..."

"My spouse isn't supportive of..."

"My kids won't eat that..."

"It's no fun to cook for just me..."

Here's a little bit of tough love.

We have to stop making excuses! Your health (and mine) freaking matters!

If you don't make your health a priority, you will eventually end up sick (or worse), and you will be no good to anyone or anything in your life that is important to you! Stop thinking you're invincible. You aren't.

If we dig deep, we'll find that nine times out of ten, we just don't feel like it. You know what that is? Laziness. Yep, I said it. This is why it's essential to keep your inner fire burning hot. There's no room for procrastination when your fire is burning. You don't even acknowledge the excuse as an option when your fire is lit up. When your fire is hot, you're confident and happy, productive, and successful. You're healthy and full of energy. You can think clearly and make wise decisions.

But laziness and lack of motivation are fire extinguishers. It doesn't take long for them to suffocate out all of your hard work or stall you in the process of achieving your goals.

If you feel yourself slipping into that mode of not wanting to do anything that you know is good for you, start with just one small step forward. The hardest part is just getting started. You know, putting on the gym clothes or chopping up the vegetables for dinner. It's a tough step, but it's a small one, and once you take it, you're committed at that point.

Something else you can try is shutting down whatever would replace your trip to the gym. So, if you'd rather sit on the couch and watch old reruns of Friends, turn the TV off and relocate to a different room in the home. If it's surfing social media mindlessly for hours, put your smartphone on silent and plug it in to charge in a separate room in the house. I know. It's blasphemy that I would even suggest not having your phone within arm's reach at all times. I get it.

Asking yourself powerful questions is another great way to stifle out excuses and laziness. "How will my life or my health look in three years if I just continue to do the same thing I'm doing right now?" I know it's not always appealing to think about potential negative consequences, but sometimes that's what's necessary to give us the kick-in-the-ass we need to get moving on that goal. For added motivation, reverse the question. "How will my life or my health look in three years if I do stick with these healthy choices and keep going?"

Finally, listen to podcasts or motivational speeches by people who inspire you. Whatever you fill your mind with will significantly influence your life, so let it be inspiring, badass, full-of-energy messages you're listening to daily. Also, hang around with people who work hard themselves and will motivate you to be your best self. This is where a health coach is so beneficial.

One more thing; if you carve out time specifically for being lazy, that's a good thing and necessary to recharge. Schedule it and stick to the schedule. You should also be scheduling your healthy habits and sticking with those.

FIRE EXTINGUISHER #2

Negativity and Toxic Relationships

In the Integrative Nutrition® world of health, life nourishment plays a significant role in our overall state of health and well-being. This includes the state of our relationships. When speaking of relationships, these concepts apply to relationships we have with friends, extended family, co-workers, a spouse, and even with our children (mainly adult children).

So the question is, do the relationships you currently have nourish you or do they deplete you?

One way to tell is to look for signs of toxicity. A toxic relationship can irrevocably damage your sense of self. It's always good to look at a situation for what it is and accept that it's not going to change, so you either need to adjust your own attitude toward that person or situation, or you can choose to slowly begin to distance yourself for the sake of health and happiness.

Here are some things that should be a red flag that it's gone toxic:

- You never feel good enough, or like you are worth that person's time or attention.
- You don't feel comfortable just being yourself. A healthy, loving relationship allows that sense of freedom to just be YOU.
- You're always being put down or criticized.

- You're fighting all the time. Healthy relationships allow room for communication that is not hostile.
- You're always taking the blame even when it's not your fault. Everyone should be responsible for their own actions.

If you find that you're in one or more toxic relationships, it may be a perfect time to start considering how you can make some healthy changes in this area of life. Your health is worth it. YOU are worth it.

Chronic Stress

"When life knocks you down, causing you to lose your sparkle, give yourself a moment to pause and feel. Just don't stay stuck there. Instead, rise back up as the whole damn fire!"

— RC

Stress can be devastating to your health, and it's the equivalent of dousing your flame with water. We all face stressful seasons of life. They are inevitable. But chronic stress is the response to emotional pressure suffered over a prolonged period. You may feel like you have little control over the circumstances. During chronic stress, cortisol, your flight or fight hormone, is released over and over again by the body.

Increased heart rate, elevated cortisol levels, and higher than normal blood pressure are all reactions to chronic stress and can lead to heart attack or stroke. Other health issues can arise as well, most common being adrenal fatigue. This is from that constant firing off of cortisol, causing the adrenal glands to burn out. Once you've run out of cortisol to meet the demand your body feels is necessary to survive, it steals progesterone to create more cortisol. This steal creates a sex hormone imbalance. The tiniest imbalance can throw your endocrine system into chaos, impacting everything from the adrenal glands, to sex hormones, to thyroid function, and more.

Chronic stress also leads to systemic inflammation, poor gut health, headaches, acne flare-ups, frequent illness, lack of energy, reduced sex drive, a change in appetite, anxiety, and depression. Because of its negative impact on gut health, the risk for autoimmune disease increases. If you're experiencing any of the symptoms mentioned above, now is the time to work on drastically reducing your stress levels before it becomes entirely devastating for your health.

During my thyroiditis, as I was looking for ways to heal faster, stress was a topic I kept stumbling over. It's so important to manage for health reasons that you can find pages and pages of articles on the subject of stress management in Google. I had to go through enormous lifestyle changes in the way I was eating, sleeping, and exercising. Stress management quickly landed on my to-do list as well.

Back then, and even now, I packed my calendar so full that I put myself in a position of chronic stress. Add to it the constant stress of divorce, emotional grief, parenting, and entrepreneurship, and there's the potential for a total breakdown in health. I am continually reminding myself not to get in too deep with things. The struggle is real, though. For me, and I'm sure it is for you, also.

What Stressed Me Out?

- Negativity and drama – in real life and in social media.
- Being overwhelmed by an endless task list or packed-full calendar.
- Toxic relationships with people who brought me down rather than lift me up.
- Boredom resulting from not getting my creativity and passions flowing.
- Not feeling like I had control over my future.

Can you relate to anything I've mentioned? What would your list look like? Here are some tips I've gathered over these past few years that have helped me to reduce and manage my stress levels.

1. Significantly cut back on time spent in social media.

It's a time-suck. The drama, the constant opinions flung around, the fighting – it's all so exasperating. It stresses me out. That said, I run a business, and virtually all of my marketing, sales and group coaching happens on Facebook and Instagram. So, my solution is to put the phone down when I'm with my man distraction or my children. This typically means less time in social media during weekend hours. I do notice much less stress during those periods.

2. Put life priorities and values first.

You and me? We have only one life to live, and there's no guarantee that tomorrow will come. Let me rephrase that. Tomorrow will come, but there's no guarantee we'll be around to see it. Therefore, I won't continue to stress myself out living and breathing by an unrealistic, overly inflated list of things I need to do. One thing at a time, one day at a time. My strategy to not lose my sanity is to focus on the five most important things that take priority each day. If I've successfully achieved those daily goals and I have time and energy for more, then I look to my task list to see what I need to do and go from there.

Here are what my priorities look like:

- Take care of my physical, emotional, and spiritual health.
- Nurture the love in my life.
- Love my children and fur baby and take care of their needs.
- Take action to grow my business and offer outstanding service to my clients.
- Manage the details of my home.

3. Enjoy lazy days every now and then.

When was the last time you spent a lazy weekend morning in bed reading? Or watching a movie or the news? I rarely get the opportunity to do that because I always seem to be on the go. I need more moments like this in my life, and I'm sure you do, too.

4. Get face-to-face with people who are on your side.

One of the things I love about the work I do is that I get to have face-to-face interactions with my clients every day. These women usually end up becoming good friends with me because I work with them for six months to one year, and sometimes beyond. These ladies, alongside my closest friends, are always on my side and frequently let me know it.

My man distraction is so good about communicating with me throughout his day; he invites me over for dinner, pours my favorite wine, measures out just the right portion size from a Green & Blacks Dark Chocolate bar (my favorite!), and he listens to me when I need to talk.

My daughters bring me great joy in these fun new ages and phases of life they're in. My youngest, given the opportunity, will talk to me for hours about everything from atoms, to the big bang theory (quite literally – not the tv show!), to her crazy, gorgeous head of curls and how difficult they are to maintain, to the kid in school who annoys the heck out of her. My oldest hugs me, asks for money, and professes her love for me as she walks out the door to some social activity with friends only seconds later. At least that's a common day for her. Other days we play, tease, and giggle hysterically over the stupidest things.

My dad and I have some of the best phone conversations as often as possible. He is often filling my head with some of the best life wisdom and my heart with that special daddy-daughter love that is unconditional and irreplaceable. He's a jokester and gets me laughing when I need it the most.

I'm blessed to have these beautiful people in my life, and sometimes I miss so much of the gift they are because I try to do and be everything to everyone and do it all well. That's stressful! But these amazing people in my life? *They remove that stress!*

Imagine for a moment how your grandparents lived. Or even your own parents. My mom lived a very stress-free life. She kept it simple. She wasn't on Facebook and didn't even have internet access at all. She didn't have cable TV, just a DVD player to watch movies when she felt the desire to. Mostly, she loved to sit in her chair and get lost in a good book. She enjoyed a good cup of coffee and talking to her cat. She cooked healthy meals, went for long walks every day, and enjoyed fellowship with her church friends. She was happy. For her, life was good. And simple.

That's how life should be for each of us. Simple. Not stressful. Not stagnant, either. I'm not saying don't do anything. I'm just saying we control more than we think we do. It all comes down to choices.

FIRE EXTINGUISHER #4

Having Limiting Beliefs

In my mind's eye, I can still see it like it was yesterday. That long, often disheveled, auburn red hair flying in the wind as I cartwheeled my way barefoot across the seemingly enormous acre of land I grew up on. With every palm strike to the earth, I could feel this wildfire of hope and dreams growing within my soul. I couldn't wait to escape the bubble of small-town life and see what the world had to offer.

I partly blame, or rather, I thank my mother for this inner fire of mine.

Every summer, on the random Sunday afternoon, I would follow her around in her garden. She would examine her plants, see what was growing, move the sprinkler to just the right spot, pull a weed here or there, and chat with me as I followed behind picking strawberries and popping them into my mouth, dirt and all.

Her message to me in her actions, but also in those conversations, was profound. I'm not sure she ever fully knew how much her simple words of advice and encouragement over garden-fresh berries shaped the woman I am today. It is because of my mother that I know and fully embrace the truth that the only limits I will ever have in my life are those I place on myself. I am never stuck. I am never without a solution. I am never weak. I am always capable of whatever I set my mind to.

It's ironic, really. My mom shared wisdom she never implemented in her own life or choices. She struggled to provide for herself and her children. She was a hard worker. Like all of us, she made many mistakes and often shared her regrets with me. But overall, she chose a simple and quiet life. She didn't chase after any dreams. She lived simply, but stagnant.

After she died, I sat reading one of her journals and cried. Inside, she wrote, "My children are my greatest accomplishment." That was all she needed. Her heart burned with passion in her role as a mother. Maybe she felt that it was her calling in life to be our mom. My two older brothers and I were her primary focus. We were her passion. Her everything!

Also, in her journal, she wrote of her young heart's desire to be either a veterinarian or a hairstylist. To my knowledge, she never took one step toward bringing either dream to fruition. Knowing this woman I loved and admired so much, this saddens me. How could she offer such wisdom, yet not choose to apply it in her own life? Was her fire for life not lit at all? What was missing? I will never know the answer.

But you see, I am not just my mother's daughter. I am also very much a daddy's girl, and my dad has no doubt been a key player in stoking the fire that has very much become my unique light in this world. The strong-minded, success-driven, creative, intelligent, highly competitive, courageous, badass woman with a magnetic personality? Well, if you don't like me, blame my dad!

Even when my self-confidence was at its lowest point, I still always believed in myself and in my potential. When we have limiting beliefs, we allow those lies in our heads to impoverish our life. They hold us back from ever taking any kind of action that could profoundly change the course of our lives in incredible ways. Limiting beliefs create a ceiling between you and your dreams.

Carrying around limiting beliefs about yourself is incredibly unhealthy. Those beliefs might look something like this:

- I'm a loser.
- I can't do that. I would fail.

- Nobody likes me, so I'll skip participating in the challenge.
- I'd like to weigh less, but I know I can't, so I'll just stick with losing 10 pounds.
- Who would love someone like me?
- I don't deserve to be happy.
- Nobody would pay for my services at that price.
- I always screw up.
- I self-sabotage, so why try?
- I'll be stuck with this condition forever.
- I'm too old.
- I won't get the job because everyone else is a better candidate.
- Not everyone can achieve their goals. That's life.
- I'll never look that good.
- I could never afford to go on vacation.

Limiting beliefs begin in childhood and can be reinforced throughout your life. Something happened in your past or in your upbringing that caused you to believe a certain way. Now you believe that this is the way life is. This is called *catastrophic thinking*. You subconsciously believe that an event will always turn out the way a similar event turned out in your past. Dating is a great example. If you were hurt, and we have all been there, you now believe that every time you get close to someone you'll be hurt. So now you don't even try. You project the negativity of a past event onto present events or situations.

If you are using negative self-talk, I implore you to stop! Shift your mindset. Believing these lies – that's what they are – leads to unhealthy habits which will produce adverse outcomes that ultimately reinforce your limiting belief about yourself. The mind doesn't know the difference between what is real – what actually happened – and what you think about. When you replay those negative events in your mind, your subconscious sees this as a new event. It's a vicious cycle of negativity, and quite frankly, it's nothing more than a self-imposed pity-party that you can change if you put your mind to it. No pun intended.

You're better than that!

So, here's an exercise I want you to take time to explore for yourself. I assign this early on in my coaching sessions with clients because everyone struggles with their own limiting beliefs. Now you will learn to use that same self-talk to change your beliefs about outcomes.

Here are your instructions:

1. Grab a notepad and a pen.
2. Write down every negative statement about yourself that crosses your mind on any given day. It could be something about your appearance, your personality, your intelligence, your employment, etc. If it's negative, write it down.
3. Now, start at the top of your list and rewrite that statement turning it into a positive. For example, "I'm too old," becomes "I'm only as old as I act, and I am very young at heart." Another example is, "I'm not smart enough." This becomes, "I'm trained, skilled, and knowledgeable in the areas which I need to be for the work I do and the life I live. I can always go back to school if I need to. I'm still able to learn."
4. Really take the time to thoroughly go through this exercise. Then take a picture of your notepad for your phone. Whenever your mind tries to speak that limiting belief, look at your photo and speak only the truth – the positive statement you rewrote for yourself. The more you speak it, the more you'll believe it, and the more your life will be transformed because of it.

This is an exercise that needs to be revisited a few times a year. If you do this and actually implement these positive reinforcements, you'll find your list of negative attitudes becoming shorter over time. Our human nature is to revert to old ways. Resist that temptation, but if it happens, you'll already have a plan to shift your mind back to the right track.

During meditation is a great time to reinforce the areas where you want to make a change. When you're in meditation, your mind shuts out all the extraneous activity by shutting down the prefrontal cortex. This is the part of the brain responsible for problem solving and thought analysis, among other things. This frees up mental band-width so you get laser focus.

During this *temporary hypo-frontality*, as it's called, you can recreate events and set your intentions using your predetermined positive self-talk.

You are your only limit. Decide what you want. Set your mind to achieving it. Then show up every day and put in the work.

Fuel Your Fire Actions Steps:
1. Quit making excuses!
2. Eliminate toxic relationships!
3. Take control of your stress levels!
4. Rid yourself of limiting beliefs

"Rosann understands the difficulties we woman face with hormones, stress, and everyday life. She understands how difficult it is to fit in everything and still eat healthy and exercise daily. She is more than a coach. She's an educator. She is so knowledgeable and is more than willing to share her knowledge with anyone. She's always willing and available to answer anything, and she NEVER makes you feel guilty. Instead, she encourages and helps you every step of the way."

– ANDREA CROOKS

Conclusion

Today is a new beginning, a unique chance to do life right and be your best self. I've given you the secrets to fueling your fire. You now have the knowledge to keep it burning hot, and you know what to avoid so your flame doesn't burn out. These lifestyle changes take time to become rooted within you. Be patient. Persist. Celebrate your successes along the way.

Eat the foods that will nourish and fuel your body. Hit the gym and carve out those sexy muscles. Focus on being wildly productive. Do something you've always wanted to do. Say you're sorry when you should. Practice gratitude in all things and love your people fiercely!

Decide. So, do it. Decide.

Is this the life you want to live?
Is this the person you want to love?
Is this the best version you can be?
Can you be stronger?
Do you need help and accountability?

Decide.

Breathe in. Breathe out and decide.

Don't wait. Life goes faster than you think.

Why You Need to Work with an

Integrative Nutrition Health Coach

More than 65% of Americans are overweight, and it's estimated that by 2020, half of all Americans will have a chronic disease. Did you know that over 80% of disease is preventable through nutrition and lifestyle? Choices like quitting cigarettes, eliminating (or reducing) chronic stress, improving dietary choices, exercising regularly, and making sleep a priority go a long way in keeping a person healthy.

Of course, you know that. Most people do.

The problem is, people don't change what they do in life based on what they know. They change their habits based on how they feel.

What many people struggle with most is knowing what change will actually make them feel better or believing that nutrition has that kind of power. You might think to yourself, "Why didn't my doctor just tell me to eat more bananas instead of giving me this prescription that doesn't seem to be helping?"

The answer? Your doctor received about twelve hours of training in medical school related to nutrition. He doesn't have time to coach you on how to implement a healthy diet or lifestyle. He also isn't getting paid from the food industry to push you to eat more bananas.

Change is hard, and it's scary, too! A lot of people fear the necessary change would be too painful, expensive, time-consuming, or overwhelming to maintain for any length of time.

That's why diets are so popular. For the most part, they tend to be short term commitments. I've been trained in more than 100 different dietary theories, and I can assure you diets don't work. They may help you to lose weight temporarily, but they are typically not sustainable or healthy to continue long-term.

The Standard American Diet of convenient, fast, sugar-packed, preservative-filled, and processed food is causing chronic illness at an alarming rate.

Traditional medical professionals play specific roles in an individual's overall health and wellness. The current healthcare model that rushes patients through their office with a diagnosis and a prescription drug fails to address the root cause of illness. It also doesn't bring about lasting, healthy, lifestyle change.

Physicians, nurses, dietitians, and other healthcare professionals definitely serve essential functions. They may not have time to educate their patients on the power nutrition and healthy lifestyle choices can have on their health. It's not likely they have time to coach successful behavioral change either.

This is where working with an Integrative Nutrition Health Coach can be very valuable.

Integrative Nutrition Health Coaches are trained in many aspects of nutrition, including life nourishment. Dietary theories, healthy living, holistic health coaching, and a unique specialty are in their training as well.

My speciaties are hormone health and gut health, and I'm a certified personal trainer. I've received training in:

- how the endocrine system works
- cortisol and thyroid imbalances
- the 5 most common female hormone imbalances
- how genetic mutations affect hormone balance
- hormone balancing foods and how to use nutrition to bring balance
- vitamins and minerals for hormone health
- insulin resistance
- blood sugar balance
- the entire adrenal system
- hypothalamic pituitary adrenal (HPA) axis abnormalities
- the impacts of stress on our brain and our overall health
- common gut health conditions and how to overcome them

- male hormone health
- the thyroid gland
- perimenopause
- menopause
  ... and so much more!

As an Integrative Nutrition Health Coach, I do not compete with other healthcare providers. Instead, I compliment all health professionals, including dietitians, nutritionists, doctors, and mental health professionals.

I help my clients develop health goals based on what's most important to their unique health circumstances and personal desires. Together, we create a viable plan for carrying out regimens prescribed by their physician. I then work closely with my clients to help them put into practice health-supportive modifications and habits.

It doesn't end there, though. Private coaching sessions are one hour and are scheduled every two weeks for as long as a client feels they need my support, mentoring, and encouragement. Programs range from three months to one year in length.

Health coaches provide a listening ear, nutritional guidance for foods that nourish a client on the plate as well as wisdom for lifestyle changes that feed a client off the plate. There is no cookie-cutter approach to working with a client. Each client is unique, and their needs/desires are different.

Sessions take place in-person, by phone, zoom call, or FaceTime. You don't have to live close to a health coach to benefit from working with one.

Health coaches can be found working in a variety of settings. Some coaches are self-employed and work from home, while others work in wellness centers, doctor's offices, chiropractic offices, gyms, or spas. I work from home. In addition to private coaching, I provide personal training services, host health workshops and seminars, and run an online group coaching program called The Better Body Challenge©.

Are you, or does someone you know struggle with any of the following?

- hormone imbalance
- increased digestive distress
- brain fog
- excessive fatigue
- lack of energy
- sudden anxiety troubles
- difficulty coping with stress
- poor exercise recovery
- unexplained weight gain
- difficulty losing weight
- feeling unusually irritable
- feeling like something is "off," but you can't figure out what
- night sweats
- feeling tired but wired
- trouble sleeping
- irregular periods
- lack of libido
- dry skin or brittle hair and nails
- skin rashes
- acne
- infertility

Any of these symptoms are a sign that your body is out of balance and needs some nourishment to bring it back to optimal health. I can help guide you through this process!

Are you ready to get started?

Connect with me:

Visit my website at RosannCunningham.com to learn more about my Health Coaching and Personal Trainer services. Sign up for my monthly newsletter to receive your free copy of a hormone health meal plan with recipes and shopping lists.

Find me on Facebook at:
www.facebook.com/RosannCunninghamWrites

You can also connect with me on Instagram at:
www.instagram.com/rosann.cunningham

Join the next session of The Better Body Challenge© at rosannc.lpages.co/better-body-challenge. Sessions are 6-weeks in length and are packed full of weight loss information, motivation, and accountability. A new session begins every 6 to 8 weeks.

If you're interested in having me speak at your place of employment, a health conference, your next church event, a retreat you're organizing, or a women's group gathering, please email me at Rosann@RosannCunningham.com with the details of your request. I'm happy to speak about any of the following topics:

- Finding Hormone Balance
- Overcoming and Coping Through Major Life Trials
- Healthy Cooking
- Quality Sleep for Better Health
- Being Your Own Health Advocate
- Integrative Nutrition® and How it Helps Us Thrive
- Healing from the Inside Out
- Discovering Life Balance for the Busy Woman
- Finding Your Joy Through Fitness
- Creating a Healthy Home Environment

...or we can discuss other topics you may have in mind.

Simple Clean Recipes

PUMPKIN ENERGY BALLS
12 Servings | 25 Minutes

INGREDIENTS
½ cup Coconut Butter (melted)
½ cup Pureed Pumpkin
1 tsp Pumpkin Pie Spice
1½ tsps. Monk Fruit Sweetener
1/8 tsp Sea Salt

DIRECTIONS
1. In a blender or food processor add all ingredients and process until the mixture comes together.
2. Remove the mixture from the blender or food processor and place in a bowl. Set the bowl in the freezer for 15 to 20 minutes. Once the mixture is set, roll into balls. Store in the fridge or freezer until ready to eat. Enjoy!

Notes:
Leftovers, refrigerate in an airtight container for up to five days.
Serving size, one serving is equal to approximately one ball.
Coconut butter, ensure the coconut butter is melted, otherwise the mixture will not hold together.
No monk fruit sweetener, use maple syrup and increase the amount to taste.

IMMUNITY BOOSTING BONE BROTH
4 Servings | 12 Hours

INGREDIENTS
1 Whole Chicken Carcass (about 2 lbs of bones)
1 Carrot (peeled and chopped)
1 Yellow Onion (diced)
2 stalks Celery (chopped)
3 Garlic Cloves (halved)
1 tbsp Apple Cider Vinegar
1 tsp Sea Salt
1 cup Parsley (chopped)
6 cups Water

DIRECTIONS
1. Place the bones in the slow cooker. Add all remaining ingredients. Set slow cooker to low and let cook for at least 12 hours.
2. After 12 hours, strain the broth through a strainer or mesh sack. Discard the vegetables that you strained out. Allow broth to cool. Once cool, remove the layer of fat that forms on the top and discard or save it for future cooking. Freeze broth until ready to use.

Notes:
Low FODMAP, omit garlic and onions.

MELON BREAKFAST BOWLS

2 Servings | 10 Minutes

INGREDIENTS

1 Cantaloupe (small)
1 cup Plain Greek Yogurt
1 cup Raspberries
¼ cup Granola

DIRECTIONS

1. Cut the cantaloupe in half and scoop out the seeds.
2. Divide the yogurt and raspberries evenly between each hollowed out cantaloupe half. Top with the granola and enjoy!

Notes:

Dairy-free, use a dairy-free yogurt such as coconut.

Want it sweeter, add a drizzle of honey or maple syrup on top.

No Raspberries, use strawberries, blueberries or blackberries instead.

No Granola, use nuts or seeds instead.

TACO SALAD WITH BEEF
4 Servings | 25 Minutes

INGREDIENTS
1 lb Extra Lean Ground Beef
2 tbsps Chili Powder
½ tsp Sea Salt
1 tbsp Cumin
1 cup Cherry Tomatoes (chopped)
1 Jalapeno Pepper (chopped)
2 stalks Green Onion (chopped)
3 tbsps Lime Juice (divided)
2 heads Romaine Hearts (chopped)
2 tbsps Extra Virgin Olive Oil
2 Avocado (sliced)

DIRECTIONS
1. In a pan over medium-high heat, brown the beef. Break the meat into very small pieces with a spatula and cook until no longer pink, about 5 minutes. Drain any excess drippings, but keep the beef in the pan.
2. Add the chili powder, cumin, salt, tomatoes, jalapeno and green onion to the beef. Stir to combine. Cook for another 5 minutes until tomatoes are very soft. Remove from heat and stir in half of the lime juice. Season with additional salt if needed.
3. In a large mixing bowl toss the chopped romaine lettuce with olive oil and remaining lime juice.
4. To assemble the salad, divide lettuce between plates and top evenly with beef and avocado. Serve immediately and enjoy!

Notes:
Refrigerate beef and lettuce separately in airtight container for up to three days. Assemble salad just before serving.
Make it vegan, use black beans instead of ground beef.

CUCUMBER MOJITO BLENDER JUICE WITH ALOE
4 Servings | 15 Minutes

INGREDIENTS
2 cups Water
4 Lime (juiced)
3 fl ozs Pure Aloe Juice
¼ cup Maple Syrup
2 Cucumber (large, peeled, seeded and chopped)
1 cup Mint Leaves (loosely packed)
1/8 tsp Sea Salt

DIRECTIONS
1. Add all of the ingredients to a high-speed blender. Blend on high for one minute or until very smooth.
2. Strain the juice into a pitcher with a fine mesh sieve to remove the pulp.
3. Serve over ice and enjoy!

Notes:
No Aloe, use extra lime juice instead.
Storage, juice will keep in the fridge for one day.
No Maple Syrup, use honey or stevia to taste instead.

NO-BAKE PUMPKIN PROTEIN BARS
8 Servings | 15 Minutes

INGREDIENTS
½ cup Coconut Flour
¼ cup Vanilla Protein Powder
¾ tsp Pumpkin Pie Spice
½ cup Almond Butter
1/3 cup Maple Syrup
1 tsp Vanilla Extract
½ cup Pureed Pumpkin
1 tbsp Unsweetened Almond Milk
½ cup Organic Dark Chocolate Chips
1 tbsp Coconut Butter (melted)

DIRECTIONS
1. Line a pan with parchment paper. (Tip: Use an 8x8 inch pan if making 8 servings).
2. Add the coconut flour, protein powder and pumpkin pie spice into a large mixing bowl and whisk to combine.
3. Using a small pot over low heat, add the almond butter and maple syrup and whisk until combined and sticky, then add the vanilla extract.
4. Add the wet ingredients to the dry ingredients along with the pureed pumpkin. Stir until it is all combined, then add the milk and chocolate chips. Stir again until well combined. The dough will feel very thick.
5. Transfer the dough into your pan and flatten with your hands, applying firm pressure to ensure it is packed. Refrigerate for at least 30 minutes.
6. Remove the dough from the fridge and slice into even bars. Drizzle the bars with melted coconut butter. Store in the fridge until you are ready to eat. Enjoy!

Notes:

Nut-free, use tahini or pumpkin seed butter instead of almond butter. Use coconut milk instead of almond milk.

No coconut butter, omit, or use melted chocolate as a drizzle instead.

Storage, store in fridge or freezer until ready to eat. They will be too soft at room temperature.

Protein powder, this recipe is based on using a plant-based protein powder. If you use something different, results may vary.

MINI EGGPLANT PIZZAS
4 Servings | 30 Minutes

INGREDIENTS
1 Eggplant (medium)
¼ cup Extra Virgin Olive Oil
Sea Salt & Black Pepper (to taste)
¾ cup Tomato Sauce
½ tsp Red Pepper Flakes (optional)
2 tbsps Basil Leaves (finely chopped)

DIRECTIONS
1. Cut the eggplant into equal slices about ½ inch thick. Generously brush each side of the eggplant with the oil and season with sea salt and black pepper.
2. Heat a large non-stick pan over medium heat. Cook eggplant in batches until tender and browned about 3 to 5 minutes per side.
3. Meanwhile, turn the broiler on high.
4. Transfer the browned eggplant slices to a baking sheet and top each with tomato sauce, dried oregano and shredded cheese. Broil the eggplant pizzas for 3 to 5 minutes until the cheese is melted, bubbly and browned.
5. Top with red pepper flakes and fresh basil. Enjoy!

Notes:
Leftovers, refrigerate in an airtight container for up to two days. Reheat in the microwave or oven until warmed through.
Serving size, one serving is approximately 3 eggplant pizzas.
Dairy-free, use a dairy-free shredded cheese instead.
More flavor, add minced garlic and Italian seasoning to the tomato sauce.
Additional toppings, top eggplant pizzas with other toppings like pepperoni, bacon, olives, bell peppers or mushrooms.

CHOCOLATE CHIP COOKIE PIE
12 Servings | 45 Minutes

INGREDIENTS
1 tbsp Coconut Oil
2 cups White Navy Beans (cooked, from the can)
1 cup Oats (quick or rolled)
½ cup Unsweetened Applesauce
2 tsps Vanilla Extract
½ tsp Baking Soda
1 ½ tsps. Baking Powder
½ cup Organic Dark Chocolate Chips (divided)
½ tsp Sea Salt (coarse, optional)

DIRECTIONS
1. Preheat oven at 350°F and grease your pie pan or springform pan with coconut oil (use a 10-inch pan for 12 servings).
2. Combine beans, oats, applesauce, vanilla, baking soda, baking powder and dates in a food processor until well blended. Stir in ¾ of the chocolate chips.
3. Transfer the cookie batter to your pan and spread into an even layer. Sprinkle the remaining chocolate chips on top and bake for 35 minutes or until golden brown.
4. Remove from oven. Sprinkle with salt (optional) and let cool before serving. Enjoy!

Notes:
No white beans, use chickpeas instead.
Storage refrigerate up to 5 days or freeze in individual servings.

A Final Word...

This book was inspired by my experience at the Institute for Integrative Nutrition® (IIN), where I received my training in holistic wellness and health coaching.

IIN offers a truly comprehensive Health Coach Training Program that invites students to deeply explore the things that are most nourishing to them. From the physical aspects of nutrition and eating wholesome foods that work best for each individual person, to the concept of Primary Food – the idea that everything in life, including our faith, career, relationships, and fitness contributes to our inner and outer health – IIN helped me reach optimal health and balance. This inner journey unleashed the passion that compels me to share what I've learned and inspire others.

Beyond personal health, IIN offers training in health coaching, as well as business and marketing. Students who choose to pursue this field professionally complete the program equipped with the communication skills and branding knowledge they need to create a fulfilling career encouraging and supporting others in reaching their own health goals.

From renowned wellness experts as Visiting Teachers to the convenience of their online learning platform, this school has changed my life, and I believe it will do the same for you. I invite you to learn more about the Institute for Integrative Nutrition and explore how the Health Coach Training Program can help transform your life. Feel free to contact me to hear more about my personal experience at https://rosanncunningham.com/changed-life-health-myself, or call (844) 315-8546 to learn more.

Author Bio

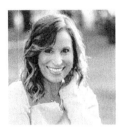 Rosann Cunningham is an Integrative Nutrition Health Coach specializing in hormone health, gut health, and weight loss. She is also a fitness junkie with a specific passion for mixed martial arts style kickboxing and is trained in Krav Maga – a military self-defense fighting style.

She is certified with the Institute for Integrative Nutrition where she received in-depth training in hormone health, gut health, holistic health coaching, over 100 different dietary theories, health & wellness, business development, group coaching, and more!

Her passion for fitness, MMA, and self-defense led to her certifications as a Personal Fitness Trainer and Core Kickboxing Instructor.

She is also certified through the American Red Cross in CPR & AED.

After a Hashimotos diagnosis which turned out to be a very wrong call, Rosann became her own health advocate and fought her way back to optimal health and wellness.

She is determined to help her clients dig deep to find the root cause of their health and weight struggles so they can thrive and live an abundant life of health and happiness. She believes nobody should be a victim in life or in their health, so in her coaching practice she helps her clients fuel their fire and discover their inner badass to meet their fullest and healthiest potential.

Rosann leads regular sessions of The Better Body Challenge©, hosts workshops and seminars in nutrition, hormone health, and gut health, and she offers a variety of private nutrition and fitness coaching programs.

You can learn more about Rosann Cunningham by checking out her website at RosannCunningham.com, or connect with her on Facebook: www.facebook.com/RosannCunninghamWrites

References

Cabot Health. Bristol Stool Chart. http://cdn.intechopen.com/pdfs-wm/46082.pdf, CC BY-SA 3.0, https://commons.wikimedia.org/w/index.php?curid=41761316

Carding, S., Verbeke, K., Vipond, D.T., et al. "Dysbiosis of the gut microbiota in disease." PubMed. NCBI, Feb. 2015. Retrieved from https://www.ncbi.nlm.nih.gov/pubmed/25651997

Chen, C. L., Tetri, L. H., Neuschwander-Tetri, B. A., Huang, S. S., & Huang, J. S. "A mechanism by which dietary trans fats cause atherosclerosis." NCBI, *J Nutr Biochem* July, 2011 *22*(7), 649–655. Retrieved from www.ncbi.nlm.nih.gov/pubmed/21036587

Clarke, Toni. "FDA to Cut Trans Fats from Processed Foods within 3 Years." Reuters. *Scientific American,* Jun 2015. Retrieved from https://www.scientificamerican.com/article/fda-to-cut-trans-fats-from-processed-foods-within-3-years/

David, L.A., Maurice, C.F., Carmody, R.N, et al. "Diet rapidly and reproducibly alters the human gut microbiome." PubMed. NCBI, Jan 2014. *Nature.* Retrieved from https://www.ncbi.nlm.nih.gov/pubmed/24336217

Dietary Guidelines Advisory Committee. *Dietary Guidelines for Americans 2015-2020*, 8th Ed. U.S. Department of Health and Human Services and U.S. Department of Agriculture Retrieved from www.health.gov/dietaryguidelines/2015/guidelines/

Gillingham, L. G., Harris-Janz, S., & Jones, P. J. (2011). "Dietary monounsaturated fatty acids are protective against metabolic syndrome and cardiovascular disease risk factors." NCBI, Mar. 2011. *Lipids* 46, 209–228. Retrieved from www.ncbi.nlm.nih.gov/pubmed/21308420

Helander, H.F., Fändriks, L. "Surface area of the digestive tract – revisited." PubMed. NCBI, Jun 2014. *Scand J Gastroenterol.* Retrieved from https://www.ncbi.nlm.nih.gov/pubmed/24694282

Hyman, Dr. Mark. "Food addictions. How addictive sugar is and an increased risk in heart attack." Lecture retrieved from (– *JAMA Intern Med.* 2014;174(4):516-524)

Imatome-Yun, Naomi. "The Standard American Diet is Even Sadder Than We Thought" Forks & Knives, May, 2016. Retrieved from https://www.forksoverknives.com/standard-american-diet-sadder-than-we-thought/#gs.16jdfh

Institute of Medicine, Food and Nutrition Board. Dietary Reference Intakes for Energy, Carbohydrate, Fiber, Fat, Fatty Acids, Cholesterol, Protein, and Amino Acids. Washington, DC: National Academies Press, 2005. Retrieved from National Academy of Sciences: www.nap.edu/read/10490/chapter/8

Jandhyala, S.M., et al. "Role of the normal gut microbiota." PMC. NCBI, Aug. 2015. *World J Gastroenterol* v.21(29) Retrieved from https://www.ncbi.nlm.nih.gov/pmc/articles/PMC4528021/

Kelly, JR, Kennedy, PJ, Cryan, JF, et al. "Breaking down the barriers: the gut microbiome, intestinal permeability and stress-related psychiatric disorders." PubMed. NCBI, Oct 2015. *Front Cell Neurosci.* https://www.ncbi.nlm.nih.gov/pubmed/26528128

Kris-Etherton, P. M., Pearson, T. A., Wan, Y., Hargrove, R. L., Moriarty, K., Fishell, V., & Etherton, T. D. "High-monounsaturated fatty acid diets lower both plasma cholesterol and triacylglycerol concentrations." NCBI, Dec. 1999. *Am J Clin Nutr* 70, 1009–1015. Retrieved from www.ncbi.nlm.nih.gov/pubmed/10584045

Schneiderman, I., Zagoory-Sharon, Orna, Leckman, James F., and Feldman, Ruth. "Oxytocin during the initial stages of romantic attachment: Relations to couples" interactive reciprocity." PMC. NCBI, Feb. 2014. *Psychoneuroendocrinology.* Retrieved from https://www.ncbi.nlm.nih.gov/pmc/articles/PMC3936960/

Simopoulos, A. P. (2008). The importance of the omega 6/omega 3 fatty acid ratio in cardiovascular disease and other chronic diseases. *Exp Biol: Med 233*(6), 675–688. Retrieved from www.ncbi.nlm.nih.gov/pubmed/18408140

"Standard American Diet." Nutrition Facts.org. Accessed Oct 2019. Retrieved from https://nutritionfacts.org/topics/standard-american-diet/

Vannice, G. and Rasmussen, H. "Position of the academy of nutrition and dietetics: dietary fatty acids for healthy adults." PubMed, Apr. 2014. *J Acad Nutr Diet 114*, 136–153. Retrieved from www.ncbi.nlm.nih.gov/pubmed/24342605

Wenner, Melinda. "Humans Carry More Bacterial Cells than Human Cells." *Scientific American,* Nov 2017. https://www.scientificamerican.com/article/strange-but-true-humans-carry-more-bacterial-cells-than-human-ones/

Willett, Walter C., MD. "Dietary fat and obesity: lack of an important role." *Scand J Nutr 47*(2), 58–67, 2003. Retrieved from www.tandfonline.com/doi/abs/10.1080/11026480308796

Staff. "Overview – Preventing chronic diseases: a vital investment." World Health Organization. Accessed Oct. 11, 2019. Retrieved from https://www.who.int/chp/chronic_disease_report/part1/en/index11.html

Staff. "The known health effects of UV." World Health Organization. Accessed Oct 11, 2019. Retrieved from. https://www.who.int/uv/faq/uvhealtfac/en/index1.html

Made in the USA
Coppell, TX
25 October 2021

64663245R00125